Jill Dawson is a poet and fre[...] poems in the collection *In th*[...] *Girl's Best Friend*, a short sto[...] and is editor of *School Tale*[...] another, au pair, writer-in-residence in Doncaster, yoga teacher, freelance fiction writer for *Just 17* and *Mizz* and contributor to the *Guardian* and *The Independent*. She is twenty-eight and lives in Hackney with friends and her young son.

Sally Feldt is a freelance photographer; she graduated from the London College of Printing in 1988. Her degree show was a series of photographs of tattooed women; she is interested in images of self-adornment and beauty which challenge stereotypes.

VIRAGO UPSTARTS is a series of books for girls and young women. Upstarts are about love and romance, family and friends, work and school – and about new preoccupations – because in the last two decades the lives and expectations of girls have changed a lot. These books show the funny, difficult and exciting real lives and times of teenage girls today. Lively, down-to-earth and entertaining, Virago's list is an important new Upstart on the scene.

How do I look?
....
Jill Dawson

with photographs by Sally Feldt

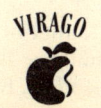

VIRAGO

Cover photographs by
Sally Feldt

Published by VIRAGO PRESS LIMITED 1990
20–23 Mandela Street, Camden Town, London NW1 OHQ

Copyright © 1990 Jill Dawson
Photographs © 1990 Sally Feldt

A CIP catalogue record for this book
is available from the British Library

Typeset by CentraCet, Cambridge
Printed in Great Britain by
Cox and Wyman Ltd, Reading, Berks

Contents

Acknowledgements   vii
My Story   1
This Book . . .   15

I Pleasures
Their Plan
1. Janet   I want people to notice me   21
2. Deborah   I like the way I look   27
3. Yasmin   How I look suits who I am inside   35

II Pressures
Do A Dance For Daddy
4. Vonetta   Blonde hair and blue eyes is not the only way to be   45
5. Hannah   Everywhere you go, people judge you by the way you look   51
6. Jo   Admen wouldn't pump so much money into it if it didn't work   56
7. Sneha   My culture affects every aspect of my looks   61

III Conflicts
A Long Overdue Poem To My Eyes
8. Helen   I can't help blaming the way I look   70
9. Louisa   Why can't I wear what I like?   74
10. Ann   Who wants to be dressed by their mum at eighteen?   79

IV Obsessions
Anorexia
11. Alison   Without my exercise, I'm a crying wreck   88
12. Freya   I'm always looking at myself through other people's eyes   97

Obsessions: Where to get help; booklist   104

Postscript   106

For Joanna

Acknowledgements

My warmest thanks are due to all the girls who speak from the pages of this book. 'Tread carefully, because as I'm sure you're aware, these are delicate areas. Please change my name and town,' wrote one, and I have heeded her advice. I'm sorry I could not include all the girls I interviewed, or all the letters I received, but each was deeply appreciated, and each contributed significantly to the shaping of *How Do I Look?* In addition I am indebted to Lennie Goodings at Virago for her initial enthusiasm for the book, and for continued and much-needed advice, input and support.

Thanks are also due to Sally Feldt for the photography, for her valued contribution of ideas, criticisms and encouragement, and not least for her sense of humour and for keeping up my morale!

Thanks too to all the teachers, parents and youth workers who arranged meetings and circulated questionnaires – in particular to Cathy at Eden Grove, to Ruth and Sylvia and Anne Rhodes at Skinner's Company's School for Girls, and to Caroline Clements at Graham Balfour School, Staffs. Thanks to Nikki and Debra for childcare and for making most of the interviews possible. To Stewart for driving me to them, and for doing the photocopying. To Kate, Debra and Karen for the hours of conversation, debate and provocation around the subject of 'how we look'. To Melanie McFadyean and the other editors of magazines and newspapers who gave me access to their pages.

'Their Plan' appears by kind permission of Sista Roots, and was first published by The Women's Press (1987) in *Watchers and Seekers*, edited by Merle Collins and Rhonda Cobham; 'A long overdue poem to my eyes' by kind permission of Meiling Jin from her collection *Gifts from my Grandmother* (Sheba Feminist Publishers), and 'Do a Dance for Daddy' by kind permission of Fran Landesman; it first appeared in *In the Pink*,

How Do I Look?

edited by The Raving Beauties, published by The Women's Press (1983).

Lastly, I would like to thank all the girls and young women who appear in the photographs in this book. I hope you like the image of yourself that you see.

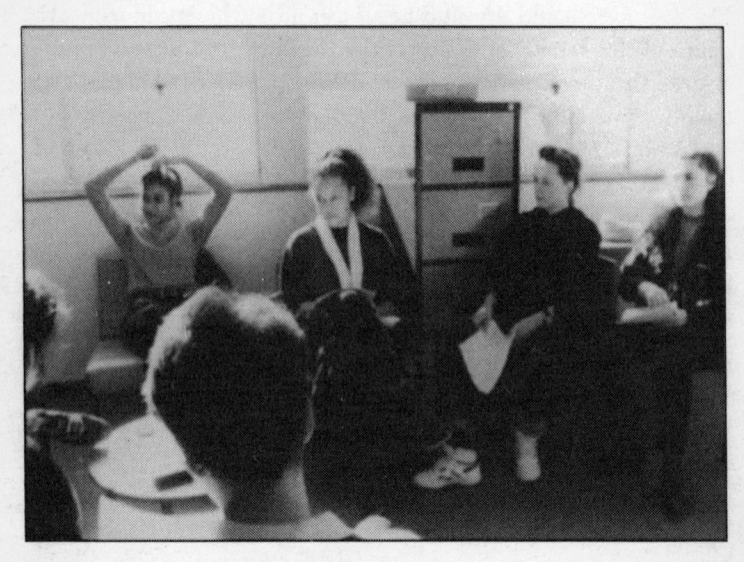

My Story

There is a photo of me at fifteen: round face, shoulder-length mousey-brown hair, grey eyes. I'm wearing a denim waistcoat, cheesecloth shirt and baggy denim jeans, and I'm smiling fit to burst, as I always seem to be in photographs. The year is 1977.

That was the year I went on my first diet. I cut it out of *Cosmopolitan* magazine: an article entitled 'Think Yourself Thin', illustrated by a blonde woman in a bikini being carried on the arms of two grinning, solid young men. The bikini is tiny, three triangles of cotton crochet, and her ribs protrude so much that she looks as if she is made of corrugated paper. I keep her photograph under my pillow, for inspiration.

I have a boyfriend, a serious one; his name is John. He likes 'skinny women' and 'small bums in tight jeans', he says. He lives on a diet of Mars bars, peanut butter sarnies, and a cake we call a vanilla slice – three layers of melting pastry, vanilla custard and cream. He is spotty, but reed-thin. He works on our local trading estate and I see him every day after school and at weekends.

Mum begins to notice my attachment to John, the amount of hours I am spending away from home, the fact that I am growing up and away from her, and also how much I'm eating. The only thing she comments on is the eating. When I'm in the kitchen she calls to me from the sitting room, where she is sewing. Her foot ferociously working the pedal, her mouth full of pins, she seems to be constantly warning, or criticising: 'How many biscuits is *that*?' or 'You'd better watch it, young lady, Pat was skinny at your age and now look at her!'

Pat is my older sister. She has recently left home, and whenever they talk about her my parents' voices are disapproving, as if she has gone off the rails in some way which they don't specify. It is either to do with sex or with overeating. She *does* seem to be heavier than she was when she lived at home, and she *has* dyed her hair blonde recently. Other than that, I can't see what it is about her that is so dreadful suddenly, but the tone of disappointment and warning in my mother's voice does get through to me. *I* wouldn't want to prompt their disapproval and anger, so I try to eat less and my trips to the biscuit tin become fewer, or more sneaky.

I have decided that control is the key, and I spend a lot of time thinking about 'self-control' and 'willpower'. Pat obviously has no self-control. In fact, the more I think about it, few people have any self-control at all!

When I reach my goal weight I am extremely proud of myself. I weigh myself in the bathroom at a friend's house, and I feel jubilant, euphoric, light-as-a-feather, almost floating. It's as if I've won a marathon, or a prize, or some huge event that I've been training for for months. But there is no one to congratulate me.

Already I have the feeling that I'm a bit *too* thin – that Anna, whose house I am at, will say that I was never fat in the first place: 'Oh, *you're* all right, skinny ribs'; that mixture of dismissal and envy she uses, excluding me from the problems of other girls, from real problems like her fat thighs, or her backside that could do with 'half an hour on a bacon slicer', as she puts it.

So I say nothing to Anna; instead I quietly join her family for a meal. I eat carefully, my heartbeat quickens nervously when the portions offered are too big, and at the same time I'm trying not to draw attention to my small plateful. I feel both pleased and terrified when Anna's mother remarks, 'You don't eat much, do you, Jill? I can see why *you're* so thin.' I sneak a glance at Anna. Oh, God, does she hate me?

I think that I'm in control, that controlling what I eat will control what I weigh, will control who I turn into. I have a vivid picture of who I want to be, and it's everything I'm not. I want to be beautiful, so stunning that heads turn in the street, boys fall over themselves to ask me out, and everyone admires me. On the other hand, I want people to like me. I want to be clever, popular, successful, lucky. I want to pass all my exams, I want my mum and dad to be proud of me. And I want John to love me for ever and ever.

My Story

It doesn't occur to me that these wants are impossible. Or that I am unhappy, and feeling insecure. The only things I think about are calorie-counting and weighing myself, and making sure that I don't put on the weight I've lost, and passing my O levels. By the summer of 1978 I've lost another stone, without meaning to, and the rust-coloured cords I ordered from the catalogue only a month ago are already hanging off me.

We go on holiday to Cornwall, John and I and my family. By this time Mum is worried about me, but she covers it up by joking. 'Look – there's someone who's *almost* thinner than you, Jill, can you believe it!' I'm convinced that I should lose more weight, then no one could be thinner than I am. That would really mean something. Underneath Mum's anxiety I detect something else, very faintly, heavily disguised. Admiration. She is worried about me not eating, she is worried that my periods have stopped, that I look thinner and thinner, that my hair has gone dry and flat and rasps like paper when you touch it, but she also admires me. I seem to be able to do the thing that she can't do; that Pat can't do; that the women she works with can't do: control my weight, my body, my self.

I am very confused. I do not feel as if I am well; I've got no energy, I'm always cold, my fingers and toes are a weird shade of blue, and I know I spend a huge amount of time thinking about food. My waking thought is 'What will I eat today?'. I go to sleep working out the day's calories, and my dreams are always of food. But even people who are concerned about me say things which seem to be complimentary; a teacher remarks that I have become 'a sylph' lately, Mum defends me to my grandma as 'naturally slender', and Dad makes jokes about my skinny legs – reassuring jokes, the sort he used to make when I was little, before I became 'a young woman' and embarrassing to him.

Mum takes me to the doctor, our village doctor, who weighs me and mumbles about taking dieting too far and makes me an appointment as an outpatient at the hospital. Mum takes me only because I mentioned to her that my periods have stopped. She thinks I might be pregnant! 'Oh, Mum, I couldn't be!' I say, but it's not true. I could be, but I do not think I am. I'm much too thin to have a baby. I think I'm anorexic.

Secretly, I write to an organisation for anorexics, asking 'Do you think I may be anorexic? Am I too thin?' I give them exact details of my weight, height and age, and when my periods stopped. I wait excitedly for their reply; every day I check the post before Mum or Dad can get to it . . . I'm longing for an answer.

In the meantime, Mum and I go to St James's Hospital and they do lots and lots of tests on me, most of them horrible and frightening. They think my weight loss may be glandular and they take lots of blood samples. Every time we go I have to wait for ages in the cold hospital wearing a scratchy towelling robe the colour of sick and drinking black coffee. Then someone will call us and they will take a blood sample, and I will be terrified as the needle goes in and I feel that they are draining me, that I have no blood left to give. Mum gets frightened on these occasions too; she feels sorry for me; neither of us understands quite why I have to have so many blood tests. One time they spill the blood. It smears my file, and I feel sick every time I look at it. I want Mum to ask the doctor why they keep testing me – what do they think is wrong? But she is afraid of the doctors. One time the doctor puts on rubber gloves and says something to Mum, and she goes out, leaving me sitting on the high bed, dangling my legs. I feel frightened, wondering why Mum went out, and what they are going to do to me. It is the first time I have an internal examination. No one explains it to me, and I'm bewildered; I feel like a doll, lying on the hospital bed, paper thin – the little dolls I used to make when I was younger. I feel that the doctors might accidentally tear me up, or that I might flap off the bed in a gust of wind and float away.

Going to hospital is so frightening that I start eating again. John is worried about me. One night he brings me a huge bar of Old Jamaica chocolate and watches while I eat the whole lot. This is great! Someone telling me what to eat, and how much. I wish John could cook every meal for me, and make the decisions for me. It's exhausting, trying to decide what to eat and worrying

My Story

about every mouthful. However, I do feel a bit suspicious of John's motives. He says that I never feel randy these days, that I'm 'cold', and that the anorexia is stopping my hormones, which he says is stopping me from feeling sexy. It's true that I don't fancy John any more. I just can't bear to tell him. I want us still to go out together, I want him to be my boyfriend, I really need him to confide in, as I don't seem to have a close girlfriend. I just don't want to sleep with him.

Eventually, the letter comes from the anorexic organisation. It's a very nice letter, but it doesn't tell me anything: 'Healthy people are like healthy animals, they eat when they're hungry, and they do not agonise over every meal.' Who are these 'healthy people'? The only person I know like that is John. Every girl or woman I know *does* agonise over every meal. 'You do seem very thin, Jill, judging from what you say in your letter. Perhaps you could confide in your mother . . .' Well, I've confided in my mother. She doesn't know any more than I do. I know she wants to help me and is worried about me, but on the other hand I think she is angry with me. I'm making her look like a bad mother. She seems to think the doctors believe she is a bad mother because she has an anorexic daughter. Then she feels guilty, and probably wants to shout: 'What would you do with her? How would you get her to eat?'

The letter is a huge disappointment. The sinking feeling I get when I fold it up again and stuff the envelope under my bed makes me realise how much I wanted it to come up with some answers. The doctors are a disappointment too, and so, if I'm honest, is my mother. I want someone to tell me what to do, how to get better, what to eat, how to stop being afraid.

But much as the letter disappoints me, it also confirms my fears. I can't put it easily out of my mind, and the gentle tone nags at me, so that I find myself worrying, asking my friends in a roundabout way: by the way, what do you weigh? I discover that I would have to put on nearly three stone to be anywhere near what they weigh, and what I think must be normal. Without meaning to, I find myself eating again, and once I start, I discover it is impossible to stop. I had wanted to regain the weight in a controlled, steady way, but instead I find myself stuffing wildly (mostly when I'm babysitting): biscuits, chocolate, great hunks of cheese, cakes, pasties; and I'm feeling more and more anxious as the food runs out – I end up eating dog biscuits, and frozen cakes and Angel Delight powder and raw jelly and dry cereal. My stomach feels as if it could explode. I have to lie down. When the people I'm babysitting for come back, I feel as if I'm drunk. I can hardly stagger home. I try to babysit for different people; sometimes I'm so embarrassed I can't go back to a place. I worry all the time in case they tell Mum.

People start to comment on how 'well' I'm looking. I think they mean that I look fat and ugly and I wish they would keep their remarks to themselves. Everyone thinks I'm well now; the doctors let me discharge myself from hospital, and consider my 'amenorrhoea' (lack of periods) a complete mystery, something to do with growing up. I'm back at school now, studying for A levels, but I spend every free period at home. School makes me nervous; when I walk down the corridor I feel that everyone is staring at me, and because a lot of people know about my anorexia they think it their job to comment constantly on what I am eating or not eating, and how much better I look now that I've put on weight.

These last remarks hurt me the most. I didn't think I looked so dreadful before, and I certainly didn't think it was any business of theirs how I looked. It's hard not to wish I was thinner again, hard not to long to be invisible, to escape all their gibes, and comments and the feeling of being on display. My closest friend in the fifth form, Mandy, failed most of her O levels, and has left now to start work. She had very bad acne, and all the boys used to tease her about it. In fact, she had greasy hair and worried about her weight too, but on the other hand she was also attractive; she had lovely teeth and something really friendly and sexy about her – lots of boys fancied her, that's partly why they teased her. Now that she's working, I'm left with all the swotty types, the brainboxes, and there's no one to giggle with about motorbikes and Mr Clarke's hideous dress sense, and the teachers' 'uniform' of one collar tucked in a

My Story

jumper, the other sticking out. I feel more and more lonely, and I can't wait to leave school.

I apply for university without any real idea of what I want to do. I'm still eating in a guilty, uncomfortable way: huge amounts one day, then fasting or taking laxatives the next. John is the only person I talk to about how ugly and disgusting I feel, how fat I think I am, how much I hate myself for being out of control. He shows me charts of average weight and height, because now he is working on his motorbike, going from door to door selling insurance policies, and they use the charts to decide whether someone is at risk of a heart attack. According to all these charts I am underweight, sometimes by as much as two stone. But nothing he says convinces me.

I no longer know what's wrong with me. I have heard the word 'bulimia', but I'm not sure what it is. Since I look, in my grandma's words, 'bonny', surely I can't be ill? And I've no way of knowing if it's normal to worry this much about food and weigh yourself this many times a day. Outwardly, now, everything is fine: I've put on weight, I've done what my mum and the doctors wanted. But inside, this time is far, far worse than the period when I was anorexic. Then I felt that people cared about me, and that I could ask things of them, ask their advice. Now I feel that I should just get on with it, do my studying, finish school, leave home, begin my 'future'.

In the summer before I go away to university I get a job as an au pair in London. I suspect that Mum is angry about this, as she usually relies on me in the summer to look after my younger sister while she is at work. I feel guilty. It is the first time I have gone ahead and openly done something that my parents disapprove of. I realise how guilty and bad that disapproval makes me feel.

When I start the job, I am already feeling doubtful and guilty. Here am I, working for a glamorous journalist in a huge house in Richmond, looking after her brat of a daughter (four-year-old Charlotte, who has her good moments but is mostly involved in a longstanding game of wear-the-au-pair-to-a-frazzle), when my

7

How Do I Look?

mother needs me just as much to look after *her* daughter, but doesn't have a big house and can't afford to pay.

Living with the family in Richmond is bewildering, and although I would never admit it I feel as though I have made a big mistake. They eat 'dinner' at nine in the evening or even later, while I am ravenous at five o'clock when at home we would usually be having tea. They think my Yorkshire accent is amusing, and Nicola, my boss, tells friends that I'm 'from the country', which makes me feel as if I'm from another planet. Charles, her husband, jokes all the time about what I'm wearing, insists that I join them for formal dinners late at night, and then teases me throughout them because I've never eaten squid before, and I don't know what haggis is made of. I've heard him shouting at Nicola in their bedroom, which is below mine, so I know that his polished and polite air is not the whole story.

I begin dieting again; I want to feel in control and it is a way to avoid the terrifying meal times. Secretly, I buy some scales from Woolworth's and hide them in my room. Charles would tease me if he thought I was worrying about my weight; he likes curvy women with big breasts, Nicola once confided in me. Hers have become very small since Charlotte was born.

Just before I'm due to come back home, before term starts at university, Nicola's parents come to visit. They are very kind and courteous, posher even than Nicola and Charles; they live in India and Nicola's father is a diplomat. Over there they have lots of servants, and her mother asks me if I would like to work there for a year, looking after Charlotte, so that Nicola could come and stay with them. I know immediately that I wouldn't like to go; I would hate to be a servant in a posh house, but I find it difficult to say this. Eventually, at tea time, I tell Nicola's mother that I can't go to India because I'm starting a course at university.

She says in her calm, posh voice that this is fine, and continues to stir the curry she is making for their evening meal. Do I like curry? she wants to know. Feeling guilty again, for not liking curry and for not wanting to go to India and letting her down, I say no, I will just have a boiled egg and toast, I'm not very hungry, that will be fine.

'Your needs are very small,' she remarks. I think it is an odd comment. What does she mean? Obviously, she is talking about the boiled egg and toast, but it is a funny way of putting things, talking about 'needs' and not appetite or eating habits. It sticks in my mind. For some reason, it disturbs me. I want to say to her: my needs are not small, I have the same needs as you, I have the same needs as everyone else! For the first time, it occurs to me that my body has needs for food, needs of its own that I can't try to overrule with dieting and ferocious exercise and fasting; and in a bigger way, I realise that I have needs of all kinds that I had tried to ignore: a need for food, a need to be loved, a need to feel accepted, a need for independence, a need to grow up, and a need for security. A thousand needs that I've spent most of my teenage years pretending don't exist, and when they've made themselves felt, so strongly that I can't fail to be aware of them, I've crushed them, trying to control my appetite and cravings in every way that I know, fighting a pointless and endless war against myself.

I would like to say that at this point everything changed: I stopped dieting, bingeing, fasting and taking laxatives and being obsessed with food. Of course things were not that easy. Something had changed, because I had suddenly realised that what I was trying to do was impossible. Starving myself was dangerous and could eventually mean I might starve to death. I had read enough to know that the figures for anorexics who starve to death or commit suicide are frighteningly high. I also knew that eating in the way I did, stuffing and starving and taking laxatives when I felt guilty about what I'd eaten, was dangerous too, and affecting my health. I knew it wasn't healthy or good for me to spend so many hours thinking about eating and cooking up plans for new diets or exercise programmes. What I didn't know was how to stop.

I went away to university and made some new friends, and John and I finished. We had been going out together for four years; he was more like a brother than a boyfriend. I liked going to the Youth Club or the pictures with him, or staying in and watching telly in his new flat, but we'd grown apart. I did miss him, though, and I quickly met up with a new boyfriend, Mark, in whom I again confided about my strange 'food hang-ups', as I called them, whilst keeping my other friendships quite superficial by always pretending everything was fine. The three years I spent studying took a similar shape to my school years; on the surface I did well, passing my exams with seemingly not too much trouble. Underneath I felt that my life was a weird cocktail of huge, secret binges and hidden stashes of food, and late-night trips to the off-licence to buy vast amounts of chocolate and crisps. Often I felt so full after eating that I had to lie down or drag myself to lectures, feeling as though I'd just eaten three Christmas dinners. Then, as soon as the lecture was over, I'd rush to the campus shop or café to fill up on more food: sweets, cakes and peanuts.

The cravings for food were powerful; I was convinced it was an addiction, like being an alcoholic. I had no idea that what was happening was my body trying to bring itself up to a natural weight rather than the unnatural, low one that I kept it at. It never occurred to me that anyone who had been starving for years would feel an incredible, overwhelming urge to eat that was both physical and emotional. All I knew was that the more I ate, the more I hated myself and my body, and the more depressed and despairing I felt of ever being back 'in control'.

I went to a group called 'Overeaters Anonymous'. It was like a religious group; I had to say, 'Hi, I'm Jill and I'm an overeater.' But I was the only thin one in the group. The others looked at me oddly; they didn't have bulimics in their group – that was a different matter. I felt weirder and weirder. Whatever I did I was convinced that people didn't like me, and that if only I could be slim and keep that way with sensible eating habits, they would.

When I graduated I came to London, again with not much idea of what I would do. I seemed to be drifting from one thing to another, trying to please my parents and trying to do the opposite from Pat, to be different. I tried joining another group, this time for compulsive eaters. This, like everything else to do with food and dieting, I did secretly and guiltily, without confiding in anyone. This group was equally weird. They had read a book called *Fat is a Feminist Issue* by Susie Orbach, and we were supposed to talk about what we had eaten and what we thought this meant emotionally. We were also supposed to dress up like our mothers, and talk about what we felt.

The group was run by a woman who was much older than me, in her own home. When I tried to say something, she told me that my turn would come up later, and there was a strict order for speaking. When it was my turn I couldn't think of anything to say. She had just done a course in assertiveness and when she was unkind (which she was often) she would say, 'Oh, I'm sorry', and then 'No, actually I'm not sorry!' It was confusing, and I didn't think it was helping, so I left.

I went to see my doctor and he wrote everything down and listened with his head on one side and a finger in his ear as if he was listening to folk music. He recommended that I go to a hospital and see a psychiatrist. When I got there I discovered that I had been sent to the schizophrenic ward. During my interview with the doctor a woman kept coming in and asking him where the party was. It was difficult to talk to him with this going on. When I said I was a feminist he became abrupt, as if his time was precious, and told me he couldn't help me. However, he did tell me about the Women's Therapy Centre.

So I wrote to them. The letter was a little like the earlier one to the anorexic organisation, asking: Do you think? and Can you tell me . . .? I received a reply quickly. They asked me to go there for an interview, and from that they recommended a therapist who would see me at her home.

I went for my first visit to the therapist feeling panicky, nervous, hopeful and depressed. By this time I was convinced that nothing could work and that I would have to spend the rest of my life obsessed with food, hating my body, eating every day to the point of pain, and desperately frightened if I couldn't find any laxatives or make myself sick. All the doctors, psychiatrists and groups I'd been to so far for help had made me feel worse than ever: could she be any different?

The first thing I realised was that I liked her. This surprised me. She was quiet and calm, and didn't talk much (I was supposed to do the talking) and she said she thought I should come every week, and told me how much it would cost. I was on the dole at the time, so the amount seemed enormous. The first psychiatrist had been on the National Health, but he was useless. At least I felt a little hopeful where she was concerned. I agreed to come very week, and agreed to the price.

That year I was nearly twenty-three. I had been 'anorexic' or 'bulimic' or simply obsessed with food and dieting for at least seven years. And it seemed that within three months of going to see her, the bingeing and fasting, and endless weighing myself and despairing at my size, had stopped.

In delight, I told the therapist. She warned that when things vanished as quickly as this, it was quite possible that they might come back. She tried to explain that it was only the symptoms that had gone, and that now we had to tackle the causes. She could not convince me at the time that anything bad could happen, now that I had finally 'solved' my eating problems, and for a short time I felt jubilant, relieved and ecstatic. Five years of therapy later, I realise what a lot of 'work' we did have to do to understand the underlying reasons for my eating disorder, and for many other things in my life, and also to have a wider understanding of eating disorders in general and what they are about.

At one time I imagined that if I wasn't obsessed with food and controlling my weight, if I didn't have a head stuffed full of calorie charts, I would be empty, have nothing to think about, nothing to fill up my life. This was the most terrifying feeling. The therapist didn't attempt to persuade me that I had nothing to fear; instead, every week I sat in her calm, warm room and talked about my family, my friendships, my feelings about myself, my ambitions. It struck me one day, walking through the busy market near her home, that I hadn't thought about my weight for over a month, that I had been eating without really worrying about it, and that all sorts of desires were surfacing – that the protective layer of my obsession was peeling away. I was starting to make close friendships, express more anger – in fact I didn't feel empty at all but full, full of plans and ideas and feelings and senses. The colours and smells of the market were sharp: the oranges and plantain, the T-shirts, toys and tea towels bright and startling – the smells almost drowned me; and every week I visited her I learned to trust her more, dared to feel more of my feelings, instead of eating them away.

It would be impossible here to go into all the things I learned in therapy. One important lesson I learned early on (which had not been obvious to me in the past) was that you don't have to give everything away, don't have to reveal yourself completely to people. No wonder I needed to protect myself so strongly, build up such elaborate defences. I had imagined that friendship meant giving up privacy, and closeness meant complete submersion in the other person.

The symptoms did not come back. My periods, which had always been topsy-turvy and which I saw as a real indicator of health and wellbeing, settled into a reliable pattern. These days the idea of going on a diet, or trying to control what I eat, or even trying to eat 'healthily', would never occur to me. Of course, like everyone else I'm aware of the slimming adverts on television or in magazines, and the vast amount of advice (a lot of it conflicting) about how we should eat. It's just that now I tend to ignore it. I eat what I fancy, when I want it. I never weigh myself. Sometimes I can tell from my clothes that my weight has changed, either up or down, but it doesn't fill me with panic or even very much interest.

The things which came out in therapy did not make up a complete, finished jigsaw, as I might have imagined. We began by talking about food, but food quickly became boring and was replaced by feelings, the things I had been trying to stuff down with food. The therapist made me feel that my obsessions were not silly or trivial and, by implication, that I wasn't either. I felt that what I was really talking about was my confusion over what

How Do I Look?

I want, what I like and what I don't like. I was learning was how to feel less obsessed with controlling my eating and my body, and a little more in control of my life.

This Book...

We are not mermaids, out at sea, spending all day staring in a hand mirror, existing only in our reflections or in the imaginations and fantasies of others. Yet we all of us swim between the outside world and the internal, trying to look at ourselves from the outside and also looking from the inside at the world, having a sense of ourselves and how we look that may be variable and dependent on many things – mood, confirmation from others, self-esteem, changing trends in what is considered attractive. This we call self-image.

In the story I have just told, I explain how self-image dominated my life for a time. I know that the teenage years I describe are years when feelings about your self-image are more intense than any other, and I wanted to give young women themselves the chance to express what these feelings are. I contacted schools, newspapers and magazines for young women willing to fill in a questionnaire or be interviewed about self-image, and what they told me forms the main part of this book. Since I was asking young women to talk freely about a highly personal and intimate area of their lives, I thought it only fair that I should also tell my own story, and set out some of my reasons for my interest in the subject.

Although self-image does not obsess me as it once did, my interest continues and I find it exciting how fashions and looks have changed; how many more possibilities there are for creativity and self-expression via clothes and image. For this reason, and because many of the young women I spoke to said that they never saw images of young women who looked anything like themselves, the book includes photographs, taken by Sally Feldt. Sally photographed young women at home, at school, in the park or youth group, in the street, or out shopping with their friends. Our aim was to show real girls and young women in everyday situations, without the false note of special lighting,

How Do I Look?

make-up or the studio. None of the young women you see in the photographs in this book is a model, and none had cultivated and practised the professional gaze we are used to seeing stare from the pages of a magazine. I hope that some of you reading this book will find yourself reflected in the images here.

The young women in this book speak of the importance in their lives of their self-image; how they feel about their changing bodies, the judgements that they are aware of from others and from themselves, their enjoyment of dressing to 'make a statement', the way they want to challenge stereotypes about themselves, the pleasures of looking good on their own terms. They speak of longing to be beautiful or of restrictions on what they can wear or how they can look, and of media images of young women and how this affects them. At a time in their lives when self-image is intricately interwoven with feelings about sexuality and identity, young women talk about how they feel when they look in the mirror, and what they feel from the inside, looking out.

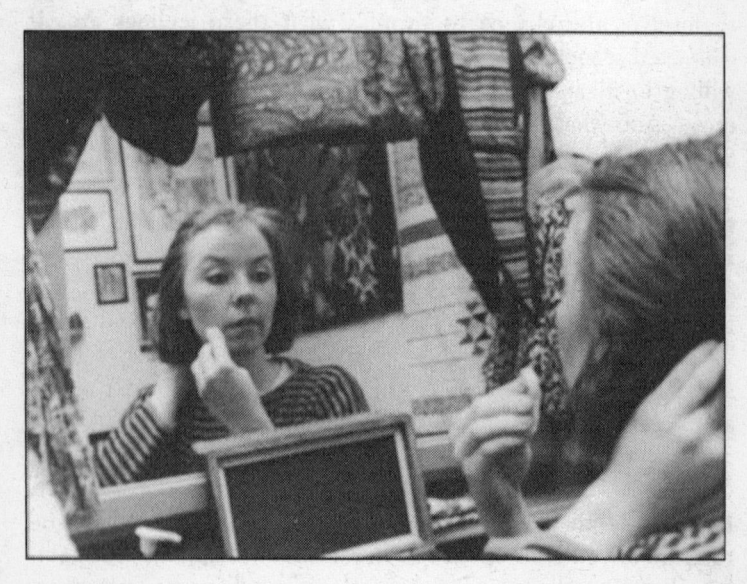

I
Pleasures

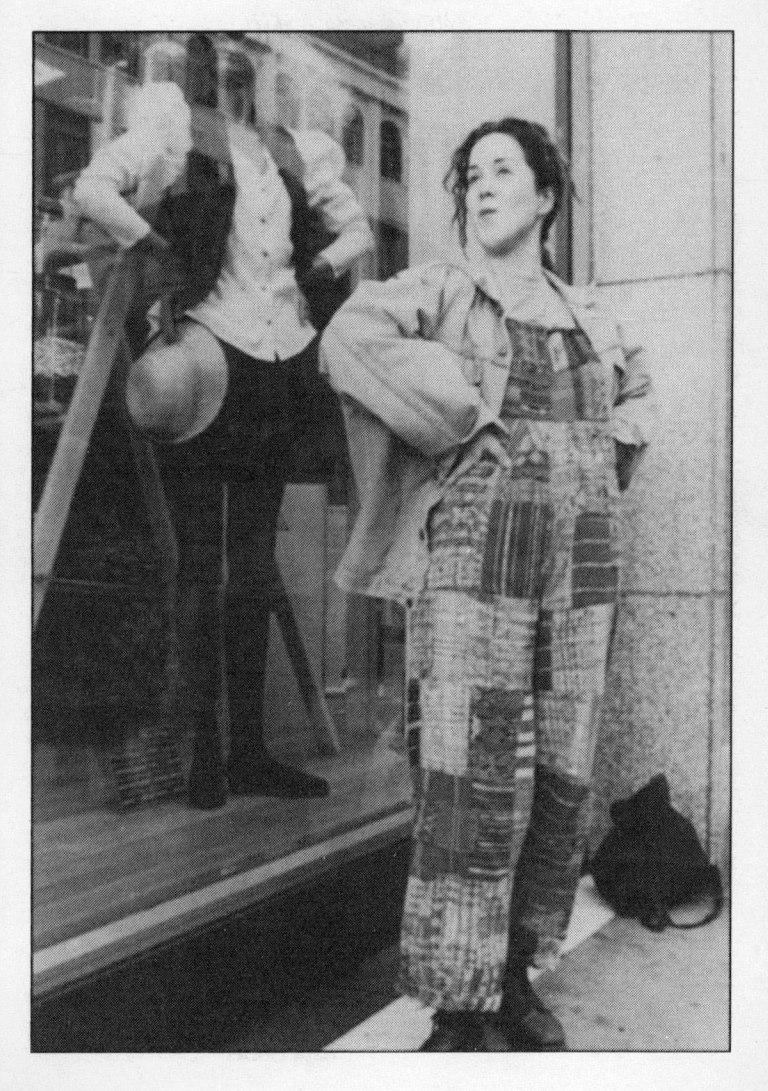

THEIR PLAN

Who says
  I should wear a skirt

Who says
  The Earth is dirt

Who says
  I should look like you

Who says
  I should do as you do

Who says
  It's time to eat

Who says
  I should eat meat

Who says
  I should comb my hair

Who says
  The best is 'fair'

I am
  What I am
I'll do what
    I can
  to destroy
    Their plan

Sista Roots

Clothes can be costumes, and for some young women, walking down the street with bleached hair or a biker's leather jacket says more about them than a thousand words. Wearing beautiful jewellery, or luscious colours and wonderful fabrics, is an ancient pleasure: that of self-adornment. In cultures the world over, women (and in many cultures, men too) have made their skin silky by bathing in oils, scented themselves with delicious perfumes, draped themselves in satin, velvet, silk and feathers, braided, brushed or oiled their hair, painted their lips and darkened their eyes and weighted themselves with gold and silver, or heavy ornaments. It is obvious that it wasn't then, and isn't now, all about catching a man; beautifying treatments, stylised outfits, painted faces, coloured hair, tattooed hands and feet, bejewelled wrists and fingers are also about pleasure for yourself, taking pleasure *in* yourself and your looks.

Many of the young women in this book spoke of their admiration for other women, other girls. They appreciated the details of a particular look, the unspoken dress codes, the way a friend or someone on the street had got it 'just right' for her particular build or colouring, and the fascinating variety of different looks, different ways to dress. Many said they definitely dressed up for each other, for their friends and themselves, and exploded the myth that women are dressing for men.

Some spoke of the challenging messages that they wanted to give out when they walked down the street in a particular outfit. One, a punk, talked about the village in Wales where she lives and how difficult it is to be different, so that dyeing her hair blue becomes an extremely powerful statement about herself, saying all the things she wants to about her rejection of the values of the people in her village. Another, who works in a uniform all day, said how important her earrings were, and the short dreadlocks under her hat; how she felt they were making a

How Do I Look?

statement for her, something like: you may think I'm an ordinary, boring nurse, but my hair and my earrings give you the clues; this is what I'm like out of my uniform, I'm different, I'm me. A third, a small blonde, always wore huge, baggy clothes and men's boots, saying she wanted to look aggressive, to get away from the things that being small and blonde are supposed to mean, and that when she walked down the street wearing her monkey boots and trench coat she felt great, confident and striding, and *daring* anyone to make a comment.

The pleasures can be for yourself: experimenting with make-up and clothes, looking different from one day to the next, expressing different sides to yourself. It can be the sheer sensuous pleasure in the *feel* of what you are wearing: how it drapes, the coolness or heat of the material, the weight of the necklace, the crashing of the bracelets. Or it can be the pleasure of saying things to other people through how you look: about individuality, politics, creativity, aggression, sense of humour, daring. For young women more than any other group there is so much scope for expression through the way they dress and look, so many more opportunities to have fun, play around with the rules, and make some of their own.

1
Janet
I WANT PEOPLE TO NOTICE ME

Janet's bedroom is painted pink, which she says is 'how it's always been, I can't be bothered to repaint it'. Her bedspread is frilled pink with white flowers, and the first things you notice on entering her room are a full-length mirror and an exercise bike, which she says she rarely uses. She lives in a terraced house in Lancashire with her mum and dad and her cat, Arthur. At eighteen she is doing A levels at college and wants to train as an aromatherapist, because she feels that looking after yourself with massage and perfume can make you feel good about yourself.

We sat on her bedroom floor, surrounded by a stack of Looks, Elle, Cosmopolitan *and* Just 17 *magazines, and I asked Janet to describe herself.*

'I'm not that tall, but I know I look it, because I wear high heels – not to college, but when I go out. My hair is brown, it's got a hint-of-tint on it right now, so it's slightly coppery; my eyes are grey, my skin is very pale, I look blotchy without make-up so I always wear a tiny bit, even if it's just powder. I suppose I look very confident; I know that most of the time, that's how I want to look. And I'm slim; I don't really worry about my body. Occasionally I think I'm too skinny.

When I'm going out, I plan what to wear ages in advance. It doesn't take me that long to actually get ready – the planning part is the important bit, and the fun bit. I'll think of the look I want – at the moment I like to look "French"; you know, sophisticated and Parisian – so I'll lay everything out on the bed, plan what shoes, what make-up, hairstyle, earrings, the lot.

How Do I Look?

Even if it's just a casual look – say, jeans, a T-shirt and a sweater – then generally I've thought it through: which lipstick would look best, some subtle jewellery. Then I have a bath, stick some stuff in from "Nectar" (we haven't got a Body Shop around here, but I never use things that are tested on animals, and even my hairspray is ozone-friendly), and lie back and indulge myself.

I think it makes you feel more confident, when you make an effort to look good. I mean, I think there is too much media pressure on us, and I don't think we should all be a size 10, but on the other hand, everyone feels better if they feel they look good; it's natural. Even in nature, cats preen and clean themselves – you should see our cat! They like to be clean and groomed, and humans are the same. I think it's therapeutic. That's why I want to be an aromatherapist. I don't think it's dead vain to care about how you look. If you have a house, you like to keep it nice and tidy; well, looking after yourself and your body is the same.

Of course, people can go too far, get too obsessed. That's why I wouldn't want to be a model. Once, this woman from an agency stopped me in the street and offered me a job and I travelled to Manchester to her agency, but they said: you'd need to lose a few pounds, and get rid of this spot, and things like that; and I thought: I can't be bothered. It's too much hassle, and it makes you *too* obsessed. It was interesting, though, to see that world, and exciting. I was flattered when she first asked me, and curious, but when I'd seen what it was like, I wasn't interested.

Around the same time, I entered this competition – it was a kind of beauty competition, although it didn't describe itself in that way. It was our local radio station, it said you had to represent them at functions and charity events, it sounded dead good. Round here, there's not that many great jobs on offer; I don't want to be stuck in an office all my life. Anyway, I got through to the finals, that was really nerve-racking, and my mum and my boyfriend came along to see me in it. I entered it because I thought it would increase my confidence; once you've walked down a catwalk in a swimsuit, you can face most things. But the other girls were more serious about it, beauty contests

Pleasures

were their whole lives. It was fascinating, I felt as if I was learning about another world. We had to hire a dress, and I was the only one who was pale; they had all got tans on a sunbed. I wouldn't want to do it again, but it was a good experience. I didn't like the feeling; it brought it home to me how much you are judged by how you look, all the time, and how weird it feels when you are talking to this compere, and all the time you know he isn't listening to a word you are saying, just looking down your cleavage. Just like the outside world, only in a beauty contest you are more aware of it!

Also the competitiveness between yourself and other girls. Ordinarily, I don't feel that me and my friends are very competitive. It's not true that girls dress up to impress men, or "catch" a boyfriend, because I think girls know that the people who will most appreciate their particular look or style, or the fabric or colour in their outfit, will be their friends. Maybe boys think that we dress up to impress them, but they will only say something looks nice if it looks obviously sexy; other than that, they're hopeless. Whereas, just yesterday, my friend Ruth said to me when I was going out: "You look great". I had a new top on, and I'd washed my hair, I was dead pleased she'd noticed. Because I know Ruth likes clothes too, and reads fashion magazines, I know she appreciates what look I'm aiming for. Men wouldn't have a clue!

But I think they could learn something from us. I like men who look good, who wear nice clothes and smell nice, and have a decent haircut. I don't know why they imagine it's "poofy" or we wouldn't find it attractive if they dressed up for us. There are some beautiful men's clothes around. Sometimes I look through the catalogue at the men's clothes, or wander into shops like Principles and look at the menswear. If I could afford it, I would buy some of their shirts and casual clothes, because often they're much better made than the stuff for girls. Manufacturers seem to think we'll put up with any old crap! And DM shoes – I don't wear them, but a lot of my friends do, and you can't help noticing that they're much better made than the shoes for girls, they last so much longer.

How Do I Look?

I always notice what people are wearing, I think it's fascinating; I'm good at appreciating what kind of look someone has aimed for, especially when it's obvious she's put a lot of time and effort into it. I've got a friend who is a punk; her make-up takes her ages, but she wants to make a statement, to be noticed. Looks can deceive, though, because to look at her you would think she was aggressive, or dead political, but she isn't, it's just that punk is the look she likes, and what she's aiming for. I think a lot of us want to be noticed – I know I do – and when we get dressed up, or put make-up on, it isn't to hide behind the make-up, like some people think, it's to be noticed, to say: Look at me!

There was one advert for Boots No. 7 make-up and I thought it was great. It showed a girl making up her face, not to catch a boy, just to try out different looks, some pretty, but some not. At the end, she pulls her face into a lion. To me, that advertisement is saying: Here's our make-up, have some fun with it. It's a bit like face-painting for children, which all kids love. (Even little boys, they like being painted like Batman or a cat or something.) That advert isn't oppressive, I like it.

The times when I have problems about how I want to look it's not to do with me, it's other people. For example, I went on holiday to Majorca last year with my mum and dad. I wanted to wear this white dress – I like it, it's cool and feels nice, it's stretchy and comfortable – so I wore it. The thing is it's skintight, and my dad thought it was obscene. He thought all the men there would be looking at me, and he wouldn't go out with me in it. Well, I stuck to my guns. I like that dress, and I don't see why I shouldn't wear it. But all day he wouldn't talk to me, and I must admit, I did get quite a few looks and remarks from boys there.

So that night, over the meal, I had a huge argument with Mum and Dad about it. My auntie and uncle were with us as well, and it was awful, no one stuck up for me. Because I'm not flat-chested, they think I should hide my body underneath a big black dress or something. But that's stupid. My mum said Dad

Pleasures

was angry with me because he "knew how men think". In other words they would think I was a slag. But that's *their* problem!

It was awful, because although I'd worn the dress all day, and stuck up for myself, I did feel bad about it; they made me feel bad, sort of guilty, as if I was showing off my body. I'm not sure what I think now about wearing clothes like that. On the one hand, I like to, I enjoy it. On the other, my parents made me feel horrible, guilty.

This year at New Year this guy threw all these streamers at me – you know, the stuff in a can – and it ruined my coat. I was so angry with him, I called him a jerk in the street, and worse than that, and I told my mum about it. At first she sympathised a bit, but basically she thinks it's because I dare to walk around and look people in the eye – I'm too challenging or flirty or something. I don't see why I shouldn't look people in the eye; I've as much right to walk the street as they have, haven't I?

I get dressed up all the time. Even for college, I put my make-up on, and I put my hair in curlers the night before, otherwise it would go flat. Some of my friends laugh about it, they don't get dressed up, a lot of them are dead scruffy, others are like me. You don't *have* to get dressed up, I just like to. I wouldn't go in without any make-up, even a bit of mascara and powder for my blotchy face would make me feel better.

It's about trying to be an individual, putting your own look together. That's what me and my friends are into, and it doesn't make us stupid or slags just because we like to dress up and have fun.'

How Do I Look?

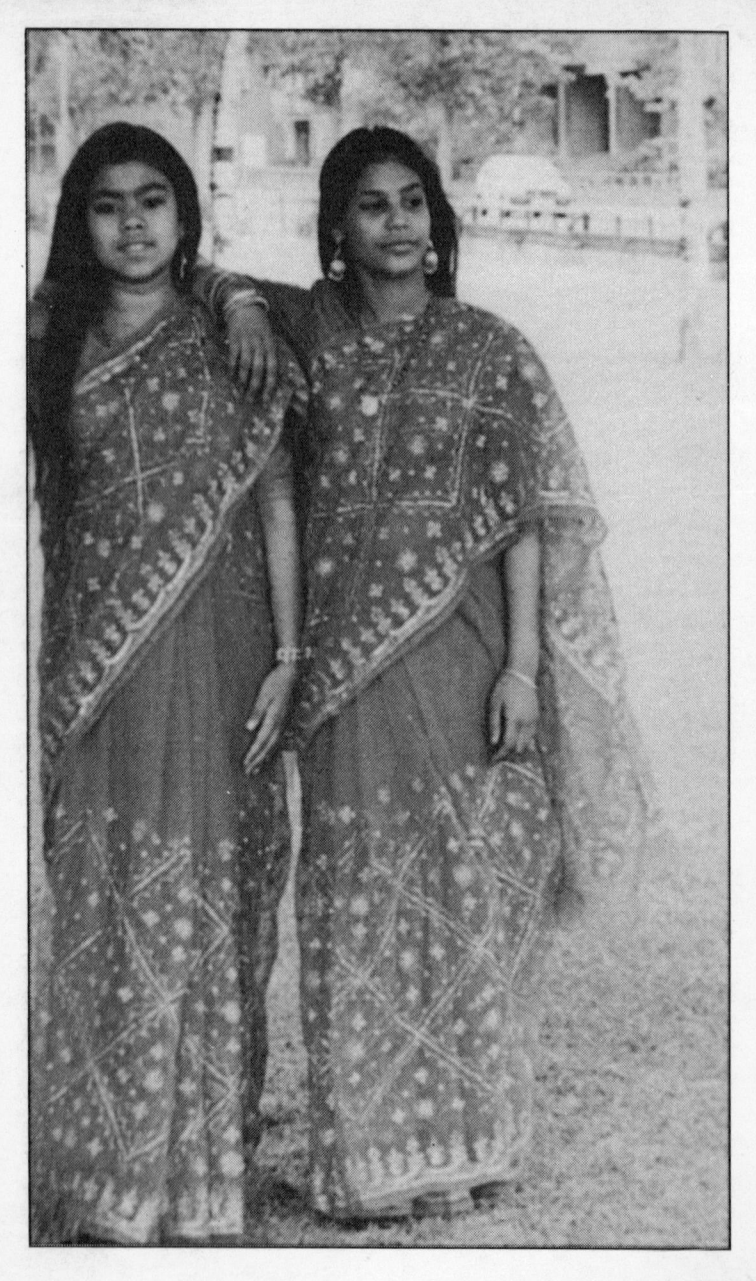

2
Deborah
I LIKE THE WAY I LOOK

Deborah invited me to meet her at home in North London, and mentioned on the phone that her mum, Elaine, would like to meet me too. At fifteen Deborah has a short story published in a collection and hopes to be a writer; we had already met whilst I was working on another book. I arrived slightly early; she wasn't yet home from the local girls' school she goes to, so Elaine and I drank tea and talked while we waited.

Deborah is confident and outspoken and had mentioned to me that she felt her sense of herself as 'not bad-looking', and her lack of any real anxieties about her weight or body was largely due to her mother. Elaine explained: 'I've really tried hard not to let Deborah and Jon criticise each other, I think that's important, some brothers can make their sisters feel awful! And I would never encourage her to diet or try drastically to change herself. I think she looks great as she is. . .

'I suppose I had to work quite hard myself when I was younger. I didn't feel that great about myself, but these days — at last — I do! I think I probably wasted a lot of time not feeling good about myself, and I wouldn't want Deb to feel like that, so I make a deliberate effort to be supportive, to say she looks nice and notice what she's wearing, that kind of thing. We don't always agree, but she's got a style of her own, and I've got mine; sometimes we just agree to differ.'

Deborah and Elaine are obviously close; Deborah's flying entrance on this last remark brought a 'The only time I know I look wrong is if Mum says I look "cute"! Then I know I'm in trouble!' *More seriously, she definitely agreed that Elaine's efforts to give her confidence had worked.*

*

How Do I Look?

'I wouldn't be surprised if I was one of very few who said they were either not bothered with how they look, or happy. I think most people, especially women, feel there is something bad about the way they look, because they get it from magazines, which are full of beautiful models and the latest diet. I think it's quite hard to say, "I feel all right about the way I look." I've got this friend who is slim, and she keeps saying she has to go on a diet, so you think: well, if she had to go on a diet, what must I be like? It's a pressure. So many girls at school say, "Bloody hell, I must go on a diet", but mostly they're not serious about it. They just want their friends to say, "Oh, but you're so pretty you don't need to lose weight . . ." in other words, they need reassurance. I feel that if you feel good about yourself generally, then you feel good about your appearance.

For instance, I've got these two friends, who are both overweight. One goes on about it all the time, saying she must go on a diet, and start jogging and stuff, the other one doesn't. The one who doesn't, she's really together; her parents are great, really caring. The other one, her parents are the opposite. And she's got two brothers who are always saying, "Oh God, not her", and that sort of thing. My brother never says negative things about my body, or how I look. Sometimes when I'm ready to go out, he'll say that looks really good, other times nothing. When I get a compliment from him it's nice, because in other ways he's cool about things. Like yesterday, when I'd had my hair cut, he did say it looked a mess before! But that's OK because at least he never mentioned it was a mess until after I'd had it cut, and tidied it up.

My brother is fourteen. He does care about his own looks, but not in the conventional way. I mean he doesn't dress up smartly, he likes wearing jeans and baggy shirts that are too big for him, and *his* haircut, now that's a bit . . . strange! He has this image in his head of the kind of person he'd like to be, it's a cartoon character . . . something about 2000 AD. He tries to fit himself to that ideal. He thinks most of the things other boys wear look stupid. It's obvious he is concerned about looks, but maybe not in the way other boys are. He is concerned with fitting his own idea of attractiveness, rather than girls' ideas of attractiveness. In the past they said men shouldn't be concerned about their looks and things, but it's pretty obvious that they are, because boys are always looking in the mirror, and these days they have slicked-back hair and fancy clothes, and that sort of thing. In some magazines they ask men to fill in questionnaires about beauty, and loads of men seem to be using cleansers and having facials. Maybe attitudes are changing.

Like – I wanted to tell my brother when I started my periods, I was so excited. Some girls wouldn't tell their brother. Mum, was really brilliant about it too. I was looking forward to starting and I couldn't wait to get home and tell Mum about it. She had given me this book, *Period*, and she says that how you feel about your first period affects you all your life, it affects your self-image, so it's very important. In the book I read about this girl who has a celebration when it's her period, and I asked Mum: could we do that? So we had a video, and a special celebration dinner, and it made me feel really great. I feel comfortable about my periods, not embarrassed. Mum said, "Do you want to tell your brother?" and I said, "Oh yes, he'll want to know." I wanted to tell everyone! But some of my friends would never tell their brothers a thing like that; their brothers put them down a lot. And I can believe there is a link between periods and self-esteem, because if people are saying periods are embarrassing or dirty or vile, then in a way they are saying being a woman is embarrassing or dirty or vile, and that's bound to affect you.

It's like the adverts that you see on TV for things like sanitary towels. Sometimes you don't even know what they're for, because the ad is just a cartoon girl taking the dog for a walk or something. They're trying to "pretty it up", making periods less shocking, or whatever they think they are. Shameful, I suppose.

But the adverts that really annoy me are not so much the ones aimed at women but the ones aimed at men. There's this one: a woman sitting in a bar, wearing a cocktail outfit. These guys are nudging each other, they go up to her, the music changes, and they're talking to her, and she says no or whatever, and then the

How Do I Look?

last guy walks up to her, the woman turns round, and she's been replaced by someone wearing the same dress but she's really fat. So of course the guy has to behave shocked, and she chases him around the bar. It's an ad for Tennents lager, I think. It makes me mad because the idea is that no guy would fancy a fat woman, that fat women are just a joke.

I've never been on a diet. Mum would never let me. The only thing I worry about sometimes is my big thighs. I think: oh, I can't wear that, it looks a bit weird with my legs. But it isn't a major issue. I think that some girls can't disassociate themselves from all the advertising they see. You see beautiful girls all the time, and you say to yourself, that's not real, that's to do with lighting, make-up, good photography. But perhaps some girls aren't able to do that, and they make themselves unhappy, longing for some ideal.

I don't think I'm perfect. I've got brown eyes, brown hair, quite a weird nose that sticks up; my hair can get scruffy in the wind . . . and I like my ears. I quite like my shoulders, and my arms are OK, except for the mole here. I would like green eyes if I could have them but it's just a passing thought, not a real obsession.

I have my idols, too, but they tend to be real people, not film stars or anything. I might see someone walking in the street, in an outfit I like, and think, she looks good. Then I try to work out what was good about it, and maybe try and copy the outfit a bit. I quite like Cher, but I think she has a problem with wanting to look *too* good. She's had so much plastic surgery done, it's not like she's herself any more. What I do like about her is her confidence, the way she wears outrageous clothes. Kylie Minogue wears horrible clothes, she looks disgusting! I don't know why so many people supposedly think she's great. When she was at the premiere of *The Delinquents* she was wearing this designer dress and it was black and cut up one side, so that you could just see one leg; it looked *awful*. Some people only wear things because they have a designer label. I don't know who likes Kylie, who has made her so popular; I don't think it's boys, or girls my age. Maybe younger girls.

Pleasures

The girls at my school like soul music, and singers like Neneh Cherry and Janet Jackson. I did a survey on the most popular pop star and those two came out tops in the "best-looking" stakes. Janet Jackson is great, the way she dresses, she doesn't just wear miniskirts like Sabrina or Sinitta, she wears trousers, baseball caps; she's more of a tomboy. I don't particularly like that word, but that's how she describes herself and it's great if people think that a tomboy is the best-dressed woman of the moment.

How a pop star looks is made too much of, though, the way some people are about it. Like my dad – he really annoys me: when he's watching "Top of the Pops", if a singer is a bit overweight he goes, "She's not going to get a hit, not with legs like that." or "Look at her haircut, she won't get a hit record." That makes me furious; it should be the music, not what a person looks like, or how fat her thighs are.

He's wrong, anyway. Look at all the big women who have hit records: Alison Moyet, Alyson Williams, Chakka Khan . . . I don't bother to answer him back when he goes on like that. He has this thing about weight, he's a bit overweight himself. Mum is always positive about me; she says, "You don't need to diet", but Dad says things like "You shouldn't drink so much milk, you'll get fat." It's because of his own hang-ups, if you ask me. When he stopped smoking, he put weight on.

What's unfair is, it's only me he says things about getting fat to, not my brother. To Jon he says the odd thing about his haircut. It's shaved around the sides, and Dad says maybe you should grow it back. But he contradicts himself. On the one hand, he says, "Don't listen to what people say"; on the other he says, "When you come to meet my friends, you better wear a hat"!

If you're brought up with your dad having a very strict view about what people should like, in a more severe way than my dad, then you would be bound to get worried, because your parents never say; "You look good enough". With me, I might have problems with Dad, but Mum is always positive, and when something doesn't look good she'll tell me the truth too. I always trust her opinion – apart from when she says I look cute, as I said! It's not just what she says about me, it's also her feelings about herself. When I go to the sauna I see these women and they're Mum's age, but they're overweight, and Mum is fitter than them so she doesn't have much to worry about. But that's more to do with health than weight. She teaches us to respect our health; that's why I don't starve myself.

The only area we disagree on is make-up. Sometimes I would like to have a go, experiment with make-up, but because Mum doesn't wear any, it doesn't occur to her that I might like to. It's not that she's said, "No, you mustn't wear make-up", but all my friends do, and sometimes I feel strange because I haven't got any. Mum encourages me to like my face without make-up. I can't change my face, so I've learned to like it, and like who I am. I know that if you're not satisfied with yourself, it's not generally because of what's on the outside, it's really because of what's on the inside. Sometimes I wear things that don't conform because I want to say to people: I don't want to be the way you want me to be. Who wants to be normal? I don't like most of the models in *Just 17* or something, I hate these jackets at the moment with flowers. I like wearing black, and mixing styles. I want to look different, to please myself as far as I'm able.'

Deborah feels she is lucky in having a mother who has deliberately tried to encourage a good self-image. Many girls spoke to me of their feelings that their mother's own self-image had a strong effect on them. One young woman, Lucy, told how sad she felt that her mother had very low self-esteem, believed she was unattractive and overweight – even said once that there was nothing she could do or be that Lucy and her sisters 'couldn't do or be better', which made Lucy feel envied and forced into competition with her mother, when she didn't want to be. Her solution was to become so thin that she was extremely plain and 'ill' looking, and that way she felt she avoided the sense of being in competition with her mother, removing herself from the battle zone. Of course this is a self-destructive and lonely 'solution'; Lucy herself admits that she has got caught up in a pattern of starving and bingeing which she is at the moment unable to see a way out of.

Another girl commented that she had never ever been told she was beautiful, and believed strongly that all children should be told this by their parents. But Louisa, who had been brought up with her father's constant comment that she was 'the prettiest girl in the world', grew up with a very unreal need to feel praised and fêted for her looks, and when as a teenager she didn't get the same kind of compliments from other people, she not surprisingly felt unloved and unattractive as a result.

It seems that more significant than whether a parent tells you you are beautiful is whether they give you the message that you are 'good enough', in Deborah's words. And if they don't, somehow or other you have to develop that confidence for yourself.

How Do I Look?

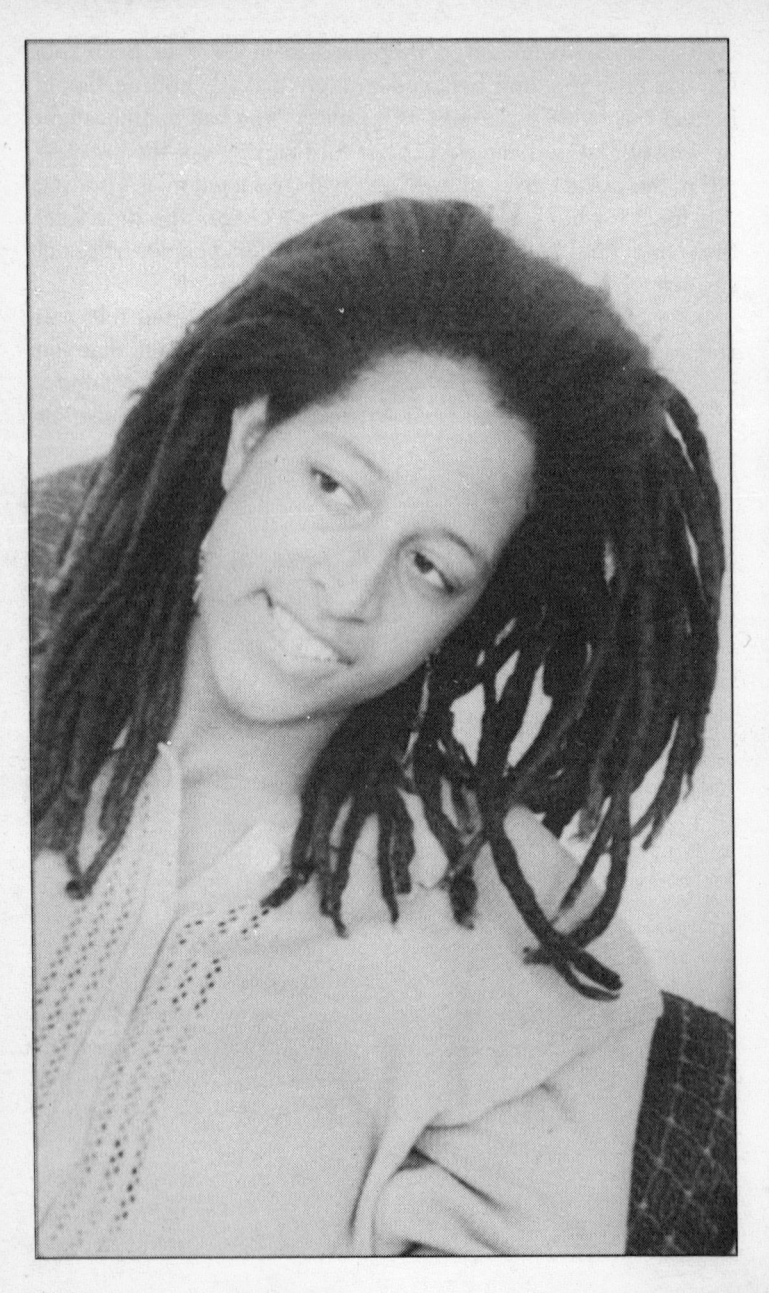

3
Yasmin
HOW I LOOK SUITS WHO I AM INSIDE

When Yasmin and I met it was Ramadan, and Yasmin, a Muslim girl of seventeen, was fasting. We sat in the bar of a London theatre and I munched my way through an entire meal (she said she didn't mind!) whilst Yasmin sipped juice, and talked. Yasmin's brother brought her to London from their home in Bradford for the day, but meeting at the tube station proved nearly impossible, as we each had only a telephone description of the other and had unfortunately arranged to meet the same Saturday as a huge poll tax march.

I finally spotted a young man and a girl dressed as she'd said she would be in shalwar kameez, a short tunic over long trousers, the traditional Muslim attire; a cool white scarf around her head and a long coat, and luckily it was Yasmin. We had talked already over the telephone about her radical decision a few months ago to begin wearing the traditional Muslim dress, and how relieved she had felt since changing what she wore, feeling that she was 'expressing something she had felt all along'. The Muslim community in Bradford, where Yasmin comes from, is very strong, and there had recently been a case which made national news of two Muslim sisters fighting for their right to wear their headscarves to school. Many religions have codes of dress or behaviour that particularly affect girls; some may seem restrictive, but Yasmin feels that covering herself is not repressive but liberating; her sense of finally feeling 'right' is enormous.

Although she says that it was not necessarily an easy step to take, her community was behind her, and the reactions she has had from friends and teachers have convinced her that the step she took was an important one, challenging stereotypes in the West about what it means to be a Muslim girl, and bringing her a great sense of identity and of no longer being at odds with herself.

'The first day I went into school wearing shalwar kameez a teacher said to me, "Are you all right, Yasmin? Everything all right at home?" He thought my parents were pressurising me to dress this way, or that I'd gone mad.

A few months ago, I went to school like any other girl. In the morning I would find myself putting on a T-shirt, a pair of tight pants and baseball boots, without any thought. But recently, I've been going through some changes. It's difficult to explain, but I know I've been doing some thinking about my obligations to my parents, about where I'm coming from and where I'm going. The way I was dressing, I always felt not right. I think I've come to realise that Western dress is shallow. (These are only my personal feelings and I wouldn't want to put anybody else down for the way they dress.) It's all based on fashion and what's "in", and that's as far as it goes. It just appears to me as very empty, to wear clothes so that you can look attractive to other people and fit in, be accepted as part of the "in crowd".

There are so many pressures on you in the West to look good. As far as looks are concerned, a lot of people are swayed by the media, it's so powerful. My niece is only little, but already she is susceptible to it, wearing T-shirts and baseball caps. The whole atmosphere of thinking in the West is that Britain and America have defined what being young is all about. That's not necessarily right. I feel there are a lot more important things in life than looking good, and in countries where life is harder you don't have time to worry about such things, you're too busy working or preparing the next meal. Also, for example, in Pakistan religion dictates life much more, whereas here it's a lot more of a fashion thing. Either the media or pop stars dictate what's in fashion. But fashion changes every week, so it doesn't mean anything.

The ideas behind traditional Islamic dress, on the other hand,

Pleasures

run a lot deeper. It stems right back from the time of Adam and Eve. Islam tells women to cover their shame and their nakedness. (As with men.) Modesty is given a high priority. But it might be difficult for most white people to understand what that means, as there is a different atmosphere in the West. Islam is a complete way of life, not a Sunday religion. Islam governs everything you do; the clothes that you wear are just bricks in the wall of something much greater.

It may sound a bit corny, but ever since I've started to wear my traditional dress to school, I feel so much more comfortable. It's as if it's what I should have worn all along. It isn't easy to change: one day to go to school in casual clothes, the next to go with your head covered. In fact it's very difficult, in one way, because people find it strange; their reactions are very strong. One friend of mine – I hadn't seen him in a while, then one day I met him in school with my head covered, and he said: "Yasmin, have you gone religious?" He'd never asked me that before, but in fact my religion had been important to me all along; he only asked me that day because I had my head covered. People see me in a certain way at school, as someone outspoken and good at English; then they see me with my head covered, and suddenly they seem to be thinking: submissive. But I'm happy with the way I look, because it's the look that most suits who I am inside.

Wearing bright colours, beautiful fabrics can be wonderful. I've worn blue and grey, the school colours, for so long. Now I'm in the sixth form and I can wear anything I like, it's great. I still find myself looking occasionally at grey trousers in shops, and then thinking: no, I can wear what I like, in bright colours. I'm still conscious of what I wear, I haven't completely lost track of fashion, but I do take more care now to see that my body is well covered, especially my head.

The reason for covering the head is not often understood in Britain. Women in Islam are held in very high esteem, which Westerners don't seem to realise. When they see headscarves on Muslim girls they think it means repression, but it means the opposite. The reason I cover my head is difficult to explain, because it's always been that way. It's not about hair or women

How Do I Look?

being shameful, it's about respect, about being sacred. You should never cut your hair. It's one of the biggest rules. Personally, I've no desire to cut my hair. A lot of my friends say to me, "Yasmin, I bet you're *dying* to cut your hair", or "Wouldn't you like to perm it?" but it's not true, I wouldn't.

I had my ears pierced very young, and my nose pierced more recently. I'm not really sure why; it doesn't have any great religious significance. One day I was in the library and I came across this book. On the cover was a punk with a pierced nose, and I thought she looked great, so I had mine done. My mum's had her nose pierced for ages; I think it looks beautiful. It doesn't really hurt, just for an instant when the gun clicks in. It's no worse than having your ears pierced. People think Asian girls with their nose pierced must have deep significance in our culture, but it doesn't. It's just like having your ears pierced – some have it, some don't.

There are so many stereotypes of Asians, of Muslims, of Asian girls. It can be exciting to challenge people's view of me. Like – the other day I was involved in this drama group with quite a few tutors. We had to work out a short monologue in the voice of a character, and then afterwards we sat around and were asked who would volunteer to stand up and read their piece. Everyone was silent, so I put my hand up. The piece was quite raunchy, and there was bad language in it (in keeping with my character) and when I sat down everyone was aghast. I was wondering: are they surprised because of the piece, or because it was me who stood up and read it? As if someone like me should have sat there quietly like a mouse, demure and repressed!

It all came to light when I travelled from Bradford to London to take part in a television programme about multiculturalism. I realised that the floor manager wanted myself and two other Muslim girls (who were wearing white headscarves which covered their foreheads) to sit together. They didn't allow me to sit where I chose. The moment I was asked to move, I knew what they were trying to do. There we were, the four of us (the two other girls, my friend, and me) with our headscarves on, looking like your average Islamic fundamentalists. I suppose they

Pleasures

felt that the viewing public needed to see a nice little clump of easily identified people, which on first glance they could decide whether they liked or not.

Of course it all boils down to image. It's no secret what the image of Muslims is that the BBC wants to project, especially of Muslim girls: the veiled Muslim woman, restricted, suppressed and extremely unhappy in her plight. It's a load of rubbish. I think that by covering their bodies, Muslim women liberate themselves.

I'm so much happier since I made the decision. These days I wear what I like without caring what anybody else thinks. But I am aware that it can be a statement; traditional dress can say something to other people, the same way big boots or punk dress can. But what I'm wearing now I'll be wearing in a year or eighteen months, it doesn't chop and change like a fashion; the meaning it has now is the same one it will have in eighteen months' time.

I realise that there are many young Asian women living in Britain today who might find it difficult to be different from their friends at school. It *is* difficult, because I've experienced it. I was born and grew up in Britain, I can appreciate the constant pressure to look the same, dress the same, forget your difference. But it comes down to how openly you want to express yourself as a Muslim. I am happy to communicate to people, through how I dress, that I'm a Muslim and proud of it, and that living in the West has done nothing to alter my feelings.'

II
Pressures

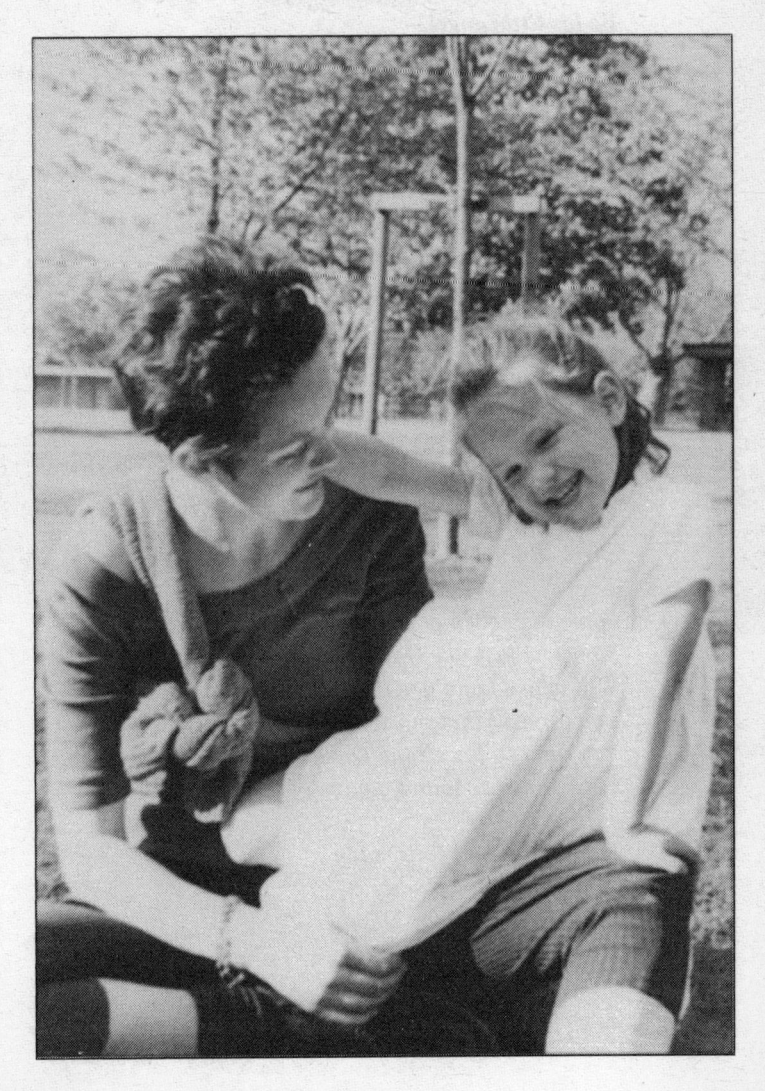

DO A DANCE FOR DADDY

Do a dance for Daddy, make your Daddy smile
Be his little angel
Remember you're on trial
Mummy's competition, Mummy brings you down
When you're up there shining
She always wears a frown

Do a dance for Daddy. Bend and dip and whirl
You've got all the talent
'Cause you're Daddy's girl
Daddy is your hero, witty and superb
With a sign upon his door
That reads 'DO NOT DISTURB'

Look your best for Daddy
Pass your test for Daddy
Stand up tall for Daddy
Do it all for Daddy

Some day when you're older you will find romance
Someone just like Daddy
Will whistle and you'll dance
You'll recall that music when you're on the shelf
You danced for all the Daddies
but you never found yourself

Paint your eyes for Daddy
Win a prize for Daddy
Swim to France for Daddy
Do your dance for Daddy.

Fran Landesman

For most of us, the first mirror is our family. The question 'How do I look?' is more likely to be phrased 'What do I look like?' and not be openly asked, but wondered about. It is unlikely that any of us could remember the first time we saw our own reflection (mirrors often form part of toys aimed at very small babies, such as activity mats or cot toys, and there are, of course, lakes, kettles and other possibilities for reflection); what *is* likely is that it was a member of our family (probably our mother) who told us: 'That's you, that's what you look like'. And it's very probable, at that age, that it was our family who told us, or implied (or maybe even talked about us to neighbours – 'She's chubby already, I'm worried about her, weight problems run in our family', or 'She gets her looks from her dad') whether we were pretty or not, and formed the basis of our self-image.

Wanting to be beautiful, wanting people to find us attractive, is a desire which is planted in girls at a very early age. I asked many of the girls I spoke to to imagine their feelings about going to an important birthday party at the age of five, and every single one mentioned dressing up, wanting to look pretty, wear a special dress, and 'be noticed'. This competing to be noticed and admired only for how you look is treated and encouraged as normal behaviour in girls. Later, we may feel competitive with other girls without even being aware of it. But it isn't easy to be envied, any more than it is to feel envy. This fear of envy may be the cause of the situation whereby even the thinnest girl will moan about how 'fat' she is, even the clearest-skinned will moan about her spots.

When adolescence hits us, feelings about ourselves are at their most intense, bound up so much with identity, a sense of who we are and who we might be. Everything is suddenly in flux; there are the physical changes – starting periods, changing shape and size, wondering what kind of figure we might have – and there are the changes of the outside world towards us: one day we might walk down the street and feel like a little girl; the next, almost overnight, it seems impossible to avoid the glances, remarks and acknowledgement that we are somehow, in our mother's words, 'becoming a woman'.

But becoming a woman doesn't happen in a vacuum; girls are surrounded by a mass of images and ideas about the female body and female sexuality, about periods and breasts, and about what exactly 'a woman' means, in our society. How we look, we are taught, will determine whether men find us attractive, whether we get a boyfriend, whether we are considered sexy or desirable. How lovable we are – or so the myth goes – is tightly interwoven with how beautiful we are. Even the size of our breasts is supposed to indicate something about us – be a sign of our sex appeal, or lack of it. How we feel about ourselves and about becoming a woman – our self-image – is significantly shaped by all these conflicting influences.

4
Vonetta

BLONDE HAIR AND BLUE EYES IS NOT THE ONLY WAY TO BE

The day Vonetta came to my flat to talk to me, she was wearing jeans, a white camisole top, and a shirt tied at the waist. The weather was unexpectedly hot, and had brought out a sudden rash of men leering from shop doorways and cars for a glimpse of female flesh, while Vonetta struggled to find my flat on the sprawling council estate where I live. The first thing we talked about was how wearing the camisole top had made her feel self-conscious, and how glad she was that she had put a shirt over it. Wondering what to wear when the weather gets hot in London is a big part of many girls' and women's daily life, my own included. I said I'd like to wear shorts and a bra top every day without thinking about it, but would feel much too 'naked' to go out in the street like that. It infuriated both of us that we didn't feel able to dress as we liked, on the basis of comfort, without worrying about it.

Vonetta loves House music, and getting dressed up to go to a 'rave'; she is twenty-two, at college, and lives at home with her parents, who are from Nigeria. Vonetta was born in this country and went to a school which had a good multicultural mix; she talked about the ways in which many of her friends, white and Black, love Black music and styles of fashion and find Black men the most attractive. It was the second time Vonetta and I had met; both times she struck me as an extremely self-possessed young woman with a lot of presence. She has strong ideas about where pressures on girls to look a certain way begin.

'I was a tomboy, having two brothers. I had long hair, then my mum cut it off and it was really short, so I think everyone

How Do I Look?

thought I was a boy anyway. When I was six or seven, it seemed like the boys had more fun; they could run and roll around and get dirty. I didn't really want to be a pretty little girl then.

My mum used to dress me up for church, but if it was up to me I would have wanted to wear something tatty. The big rage then (the seventies) was long dresses. I had two long dresses, a summer one and a winter one. It seemed a treat to put a long dress on, I actually enjoyed it; but to play around in I had jeans and trousers, so I had the best of both worlds really.

The only thing I wanted was long hair. I used to put a mop on my head and pretend it was my hair. I think the reason I wanted long hair was because all my dolls were Sindys and Pippas, and they all had long blonde hair, so that was what I wanted. When I put the mop on my head, I didn't want dreadlocks, I wanted blonde hair like Sindy's. Barbie, Pippa, Sindy, baby dolls – I had all of them. I wanted the doll with the hair that grows, too, but I don't think I had that one. I had only one Black doll when I was little. The figures on those dolls – the Barbies especially – were ridiculous! Huge busts and ridiculous waists that no one could possibly have.

But you tend to think that's what a girl should look like – blonde hair and blue eyes – and then you look in the mirror and you've got short Afro hair, and that's when you maybe start thinking that's the only way to be. I think it's only due to the way I was brought up by my mum that I didn't grow up with this real block, thinking it's great to be white. Because my mum took the trouble to buy a Black doll. Unlike now, when it's easy to buy Black dolls, then it was very difficult. I have a niece; they didn't have any problem finding Black dolls for her, and nowadays you do see some Black people on TV too, whereas when I was a kid, that was very unusual.

When I went to junior school it was half and half, white and Black kids; the Black guys were really revered, and lots of the white boys would try to act Black, because they associated it with being hard or cool. Down my way Blacks are seen as cool and trendy, especially with Acid House music, which has brought a lot of races together. Before you'd go to a rave and it would be: only Black people go to that rave, only white people go to that rave; now it's merged. White people who live in an area like Neasden, Dalston, wherever, should really be talking about how much Black culture influences them, instead of it being always us who have to talk about the influences of white culture on us. I've got this white friend who grew up in Stoke Newington, and she really loves Reggae, she knows everything about it. She doesn't try to *be* Black, but she appreciates Black culture, Black fashion.

It's like white people make these generalisations about our culture, without really understanding it. People say, for instance, that it's more acceptable in Jamaican cultures for the women to be fatter. You've got to remember that this is in Jamaica, and we're in England. And also you've got to remember that it might be OK for Jamaican or West Indian or African women to be bigger when they're older, but most of them were slim when they were young. My mum was. She's the fifties or sixties generation, and then it was all slimness, tight dresses. It might be more acceptable when you're older, when you've had a few kids, to be fatter. When you're young, in every culture, you try to look whatever is in style at that moment. The fifties was a fuller-figured look, but the sixties, that was Twiggy – she's got a lot to answer for. Ever since then, being thin has been in and it's still here today.

My generation, who are usually born here, are influenced by the culture here. If you're Irish or Polish, no one can tell by your skin, they can only tell by your name. But if you're Black, you stand out already, so you try, from a very young age, to seem as acceptable as possible. And if being thin is more acceptable than being fat, then of course Black girls will want to be thin.

Every culture in Britain at the moment has a similar philosophy as far as size goes: if you want to look good, be desirable, you've got to be thin. If you go into any of the high-street shops, and try and get something decent over a size 14, there's no way you can do it, unless you want to make your own clothes. The trouble is, a lot of girls will never be thin; it's just not natural to

How Do I Look?

them. When I was young I was like a stick insect, then at fourteen or fifteen I put on weight. I was eating cakes in the morning before I went to school and for about two years I was dieting, trying one diet or another. Then I seemed to grow a couple of inches, and thin out.

Although I've said I'm happy with how I look, it doesn't mean there's nothing about myself I wouldn't like to change. I know I'm not the ugliest person in the world, but then again, I don't want to walk around thinking I'm the prettiest, I'm perfect, I don't need to change a thing. I suppose that might be a fear of being considered big-headed or vain. You read in magazines that even top models are often unhappy with their looks, and it's true that the pressures on us mean we are never allowed to feel all right about ourselves. On the other hand, that model might be saying that so that she doesn't have the envy of thousands of women heaped on her head! Sometimes you daren't say yes, I like the way I look, because you're afraid that somebody will judge you harshly: Why are you happy with the way you look, you've got short mousey brown hair? or whatever. I try to be a bit middle-of-the-road, saying yes, I'm not particularly bothered about how I look. It's covering myself, really, asking people to take me as they find me. If they think I'm pretty, that's nice, I'm complimented; but if they don't think I am, I haven't put myself on the line.

Aiming for perfection is all down to the influence of the media. It's changed how we think about ourselves. If someone like a model says yes, I'm gorgeous, we can all pick on her for that, saying, oh yes she's got those looks, but what a horrible person. When she puts herself down, we can accept her. We might say, Jerry, what are you worrying for – you're beautiful! We don't see it as a bad quality in women to put themselves down, we see it as a good one. It isn't seen as a feminine quality, confidence; girls are supposed to be quite demure. If a girl at school was very confident, we would just think she was really "extra" – who does she think she is? It's men who are complimented for being "cocky", who thrive on that kind of vanity and self-assurance.

With men, there's a lot more possibilities for respect. You can

Pressures

be a sex symbol when you're sixty-five; there are film stars like Paul Newman whom women still think are gorgeous. With women I can't think of any examples of that. There's a lot less emphasis on men to be stunning, it's all about power and whether they can do their job. Even in the acting profession women like Glenda Jackson don't get the acclaim they deserve, because they aren't particularly pretty.

There again, being "pretty" can be one big hassle. I wasn't the sort of girl when I was younger that men lean out of cars and shout things to, and I'm glad. Sometimes you feel in summer that you have to go around in jeans rather than wear shorts and suffer the hassle you get. Some guy might walk past and say, "Hey, you look nice today", and leave it at that. That I think of as a compliment, and it makes me feel good. But if someone goes past and says, "Hey, look at you – sexy!" then that's horrible, a real pain, you feel self-conscious. Last year, a judge said there were more car accidents in summer because men were watching girls in short skirts! That's their problem, if they can't keep their eyes on the road.

Imagine if you walked down a street and said to a man, "Hey, I like your hair", or "You look nice today". They'd think: I know what *you* want, because girls are not expected to take the initiative. Just the same as, if you have a big bust, you are seen as stupid, or a dolly bird, or even a sex-crazy woman. Your bust is one of the sexual features, and it's really out front, so it's embarrassing. Men might say, "She's got a nice pair." No one would ever go up to a man and comment on what's in his trousers!

It can be horrible if you have a huge bust. I'd never wear anything clingy; I might wear a camisole, like this, but I'd put a shirt over it before I went out. You read in the papers all the time about girls being raped and murdered, and you don't want it to happen to you, so you try to cut down the odds. It's as if we're taking responsibility for men's problem, but if I want to be safe, I feel I have to.

If someone could wave a magic wand, and I could change something, I think I'd like to go down a couple of cup sizes.

How Do I Look?

Even though I've accepted myself, it doesn't mean I wouldn't want to look better sometimes. But on the whole, I feel I've spent too many years trying to be other people. I've just come to realise: this is my life, I don't know how long I've got, I might as well enjoy that time being me, because I'm stuck with this body, this face, this skin colour; I have to make the most of it. I don't see the point of being unhappy.'

5
Hannah

EVERYWHERE YOU GO, PEOPLE JUDGE YOU BY THE WAY YOU LOOK

Hannah is eighteen and lives on her own in a bedsit in Staffordshire, where she is training to be a vet. She wrote to me about the many pressures on girls to worry constantly about their looks, and in particular their bodies. She identifies advertising as one of the main forms of these, and feels that the pressure is intensified by the attitudes of friends and family who have been influenced by the media and make it extremely difficult for girls to remain impervious to the images of beauty which surround them: on TV, in films, magazines and newspapers.

'There is definitely an "ideal girl", and I've nothing to do with the creation of her. She is whatever the majority of men regard as sexy at any given moment. With all this yuppie rubbish at the moment, I'd say it's long hair, neat but sexy clothes, of course long nails, straight teeth, small nose, big eyes, shaved armpits and legs, nice perfume, and an independent-but-dying-to-be-subservient look about her. That's what the admen are promoting right now.

Naturally, I'm dissatisfied with how I look, not because I'm stupid and impressionable but because so many images of beautiful young women around make me feel self-conscious, constantly aware of myself. It's not that I *want* to be the ideal woman; I'd simply like to be able to walk down a street and not even think about it. Maybe if I could make myself invisible, then I could walk down a street without feeling on trial for the way I look.

I know that girls in magazines are not real, in the sense that it's the make-up artist, fashion adviser, photographer and stylist who have created them. They don't *look* real, anyway; they are all thin, spotless, and they obviously don't do anything practical (like walk around, for instance). The other strange thing is that they look happy all the time. All the same, they depress me. I end up wanting to look thinner; I'd like to have a big nose because I am fed up with people telling me mine is "cute"; I'd like to have naturally dark eyebrows and eyelashes, so I wouldn't look like a heroin addict without any make-up on; straighter teeth, no spots and a better haircut. The list is endless! Also I'd like to be taller and be able to afford to spend more money on clothes that would "express my personality".

In fact, money has a lot to do with it. If you have a lot of money, you can "buy" beauty. You can afford to have your teeth done, a false tan, your hair done at Vidal Sassoon. We've never had much money in our family. People are always asking me why I dress strangely, or saying, "What does your mother think of your outfits?" A lot of my clothes are holey, and if I had more money I definitely would dress quite differently. Not that I want to look as if I shop at Next, or look cute, or anything, it's just that I can't afford to dress the way I'd like to.

Luckily, my mum is sound; she never would have thrown me out for putting rips in my jeans or anything like that. I've got a friend who recently dyed her hair purple because everyone knows you aren't going to get a decent – not to mention interesting – job with a "punky" hairstyle, pierced nose and scruffy clothes, and she wants to stay in college. That just goes to show how much people judge each other on how they look. It's not the same for boys, they are respected more in society. Men don't think they have to try hard to attract women, because the women are out there falling over themselves trying to become "perfect" for the men. There is little, if any, social pressure on men to make themselves attractive to women. Boys seem to make an effort only if they are going into a situation where they know they might meet someone they fancy, whereas lots of girls I know will put on make-up just to go to the local shop! They are told by the media, and everything else, that their main function in life is to be attractive.

It makes me incredibly angry to think what a brainless, totally impossible, "perfect" image of womanhood the media present, and that so many of us, me included, are intelligent but can't seem to separate ourselves from wanting those ideals. Loads of my friends are miserable over the way they look, and the media are basically saying, "Yes, you're right to be miserable. Why aren't you perfect?" It's reinforced everywhere you go. Complete strangers in the street – men – will give you detailed descriptions of their opinions on how you look. I'm not going to stop dressing the way I want to just because they don't like it, but it's discouraging.

Even my dad, he makes sexist remarks to me about my looks. He's a sexist jerk anyway, I've never lived with him. He thinks all women should look like Page 3 models, so he always comments on my short haircut, clumpy shoes, "man's" coat, etc. He takes little interest in me apart from how I look and what my exam results are like. Luckily I only see him one to three times a year – when I need money usually.

When I lived at home my mum was cool about whatever I wore; her only considerations were practical ones, like insisting I wore ten million jumpers if I went out in the cold. But she does hassle me to eat, especially when I'm in her house. She runs through everything she's got in, until she can find something I want. Sometimes I'm really embarrassed about eating in front of people, in case they think I'm greedy or fat. When I was younger I thought I was fat, even though I was actually skinny, looking at photos. Now, I don't understand how I could ever have thought I was fat. I think I was just miserable, and it was far easier to believe the reason was something I could do something about, rather than face the fact that my depression was very complicated, based on things like my family not having much money, and feeling very isolated and different from the kids at school.

It improved when I made this close friend, who had some of the same ideas as me on things like sex, drugs, politics, music. My mum had always been very open, but I had problems talking to her simply because she was my mum. Like – when I started my period she said, "Congratulations, now you're a woman", but then it was all this hassle about hiding your sanitary towels and tampons from boys, and living in mortal fear that they would fall out of your bag and boys would know it was your period.

When you think of the adverts for tampons and towels, you can see why girls feel such a mixture of pride and shame. Tampon adverts are saying things like: use our product, and you can pretend periods don't exist. You can go out with your boyfriend without feeling embarrassed. So the idea is that you have to pretend not to have periods, deny their existence. And what kind of relationship can you have, if you daren't even tell your boyfriend you're on a period?

It's considered disgusting to use Lilets, because of the idea that the female body itself is disgusting, and that touching yourself is the equivalent of masturbation. My mum was always saying, "Masturbation's fun! It's good for you!" so I didn't have those kind of hang-ups. But I knew better than to broadcast those ideas around school.

The Tampax advert isn't the only one that makes me angry. There's the Flake one, which promotes the idea that chocolate gives you sexual gratification – and that girls who consume chocolate all day are thin and have perfect skin and teeth. I think it's all lies! My ideal would be to not give a damn as much as possible. To try and do what makes me happy, dress in a way that makes me happy. This gets distorted, though; for instance, living on chocolate makes me happy, but so does not getting spots or flab. My mum always tells me I'm the most beautiful woman in the world; she told me this even when I had chickenpox!'

Pressures

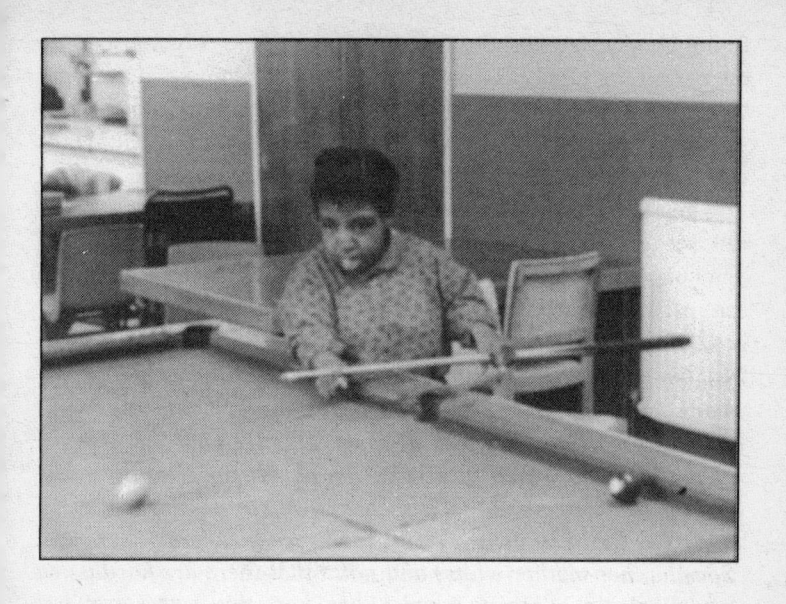

6
Jo

ADMEN WOULDN'T PUMP SO MUCH MONEY INTO IT IF IT DIDN'T WORK

Studying advertising at college in her media studies course has made Jo, who is twenty-two, aware of how television and magazine advertising affect all of us. Like Hannah she is angry at the ideal presented to her by the advertising world, as she feels it has nothing to do with her, yet still has the power to make her feel dissatisfied. Jo is mixed race (her father was from Somalia, her mother white) and notes that there are hardly any media images of young women like her; this makes her feel invisible, but angry. When she was younger her summer tan drew abusive comments like 'Paki', and she learned how differently people behaved to her when they were unaware of her race (in winter her skin can be quite pale). She thinks that more images of Black and Asian girls in the media would help to change some of the racist ideas and stereotypes that exist.

Jo's lesbianism is also important to the way she dresses; she doesn't want to look what she calls 'too femme', and says that when she wears a skirt she gets a lot more hassle from men. She prefers the sports look. The day we met she wore trainers, tracksuit bottoms and a striped loose top; her shoulder-length curly hair was in a pony tail beneath a neat African-style hat. Despite recognising the power of the advertising world, Jo does feel that there is some possibility for girls to pick and choose between what is offered to them by the media, and how they want to look themselves.

'Most ads, unless they are domestic ones for washing powder or food, are directed at girls under twenty-five. Hairspray, make-up, fashion clothes, magazines – all those ads show white, young, slender people and nothing else. Even the ones that aren't *about* image include image – like the Coke advert, for instance. The whole scene is made to look erotic, romantic, all these young types – what's that got to do with a can of Coke? Basically, girls and women are used to sell things. The model you see is secondary; she is there to sell the product. That's what I find so insulting: they are constantly using us to sell things.

The ad people know that girls are watching and that they can attract them and form their ideas by making the girl associate their product with a particular image – so that when she is looking at a hair gel in a chemist's, that will conjure up for her the image of the model used to advertise it, and make her want to look that way herself, and want to buy it. The trouble is, those images don't just *appeal* to girls, they give them complexes about themselves; worrying about what they should look like, act like, talk like, walk like. Using girls entices both sexes to use the product. Men think (subconsciously): buy the product, get the girl. Women think: buy the product, look like that. We can all think that we're not that gullible or stupid; for instance, I buy most of my things, shampoo and stuff at the Body Shop (which doesn't advertise that way) because I'm a vegetarian and I don't believe in animal testing. But on the other hand, there are always *some* things – chocolate ads, for instance – that seduce me. Have you noticed how so many adverts for chocolate are aimed at girls? They promise romance, sex, fun . . . the Bounty ad, for instance. It is a kind of brainwashing, because underneath the ad for the chocolate is another kind of message, saying you must be slim, heterosexual, white; you have to be a certain class, have money. It's all done in a few seconds, which means it's even harder for you to fend off the messages; they go in subliminally, which means you aren't aware of them.

At college, I did this project on images of Black women in the media, because it bothered me. I thought: we live in a multicultural society, but everything we see is white and stereotyped. Adverts are supposed to be showing you real life, but where's *my* life and *my* experiences? I can only think of two adverts with Black children on. There was that one for Pepsi a while back

How Do I Look?

with a little boy and a famous Black American baseball player. That's the other thing. Black people in the media are always either pop stars or sports people, or else really glamorous. So you don't see any real Black girls, what they look like.

There's that other one, for Abbey National. It's a load of children around the piano, and one little girl is mixed race, and she is stunningly beautiful, and I think: what's some old guy playing the piano surrounded by beautiful half-dressed little children got to do with Abbey National? I hate that ad. Worse than that, in a way, was the butter one a while back. It showed a little girl with a garland around her neck, and a grass skirt, on an island, being spied on by this little boy through a telescope. With all this child sex abuse going on, why show a little girl in such a sexy, provocative way? It's horrible.

Some people might say advertising reflects society, but I think it can be the other way round. I think adverts can create society, create the values and the things we want. I know women are involved in the business, but they are just toeing the line, repeating the same old images, playing the men's game. If they got together and started to change things, showing real women or girls, then things could start to alter. Like – I'd like to see an advert with a really big woman trying on a pair of jeans. Big women can wear jeans, so why do they never show it? That would be great.

Another argument is that advertising has only been around for a while, so how can that be the reason for all our hang-ups, but that's not true either. There's been advertising for years, not just since the fifties; there was advertising in Victorian times; newspapers and magazines, and pornography with drawings of women, and how men thought women should look, and the theatre and books all put out the same sorts of things – this is how a woman should be.

Like – if you said to an adman: use some real people, use me or my friends in your ad, they would say: it won't sell. It's all about fantasy, selling you a dream, things you don't have (like beauty, or money, or white skin) but want to have. The glamour adverts are about what they think we *want* to be, then there are the other kind that are supposedly about reality – you know, the ones where they always have Northern accents. They're for things like spot cream. For instance, there's one where two girls watch their brothers playing football and one's got a bucket on his head. Or the two girls and one is a greaser until she tries this spot cream and suddenly she turns into this total straight. Yuk! That's saying that being a biker or a greaser or a punk is dirty – that's a real stereotype old people believe about young people. Those spot-cream adverts are to make you feel ashamed of yourself. They're saying: if you've got spots, cover your face. If you're not beautiful in our image, then put a bucket over your head, or hide at home if you're too fat; we don't want to see you.

I think all women are obsessed with something, and it's due to the media. I'm obsessed with my weight, even though I know I'm not fat. I know some women who are big and they think they look great, but I can't feel like that. I like the way I dress, though, I've always had this thing for a sports look, that's what I'm aiming for. Tracksuit bottoms, trainers, loose tops. And labels, I do notice labels. Like – if I was wearing jeans it would only be 501s and that kind of thing. I've been into this look for quite a while now, I know the rules. The silly thing is that the labels only matter to you if you do know the rules yourself. If I went into a club or something, I would notice other people's clothes, and the label, even though I think it's silly in a way, and I know they'd notice mine.

I think it's a class thing. I've lived in the East End all my life; there is a certain look here, especially for young Black girls, and I like it, it's very comfortable. The clothes are for comfort, for running and moving, not just for looking good. I can imagine looking like this, having this image, until I'm forty. I think it's what I'm aiming for, what I want to say about myself.'

How Do I Look?

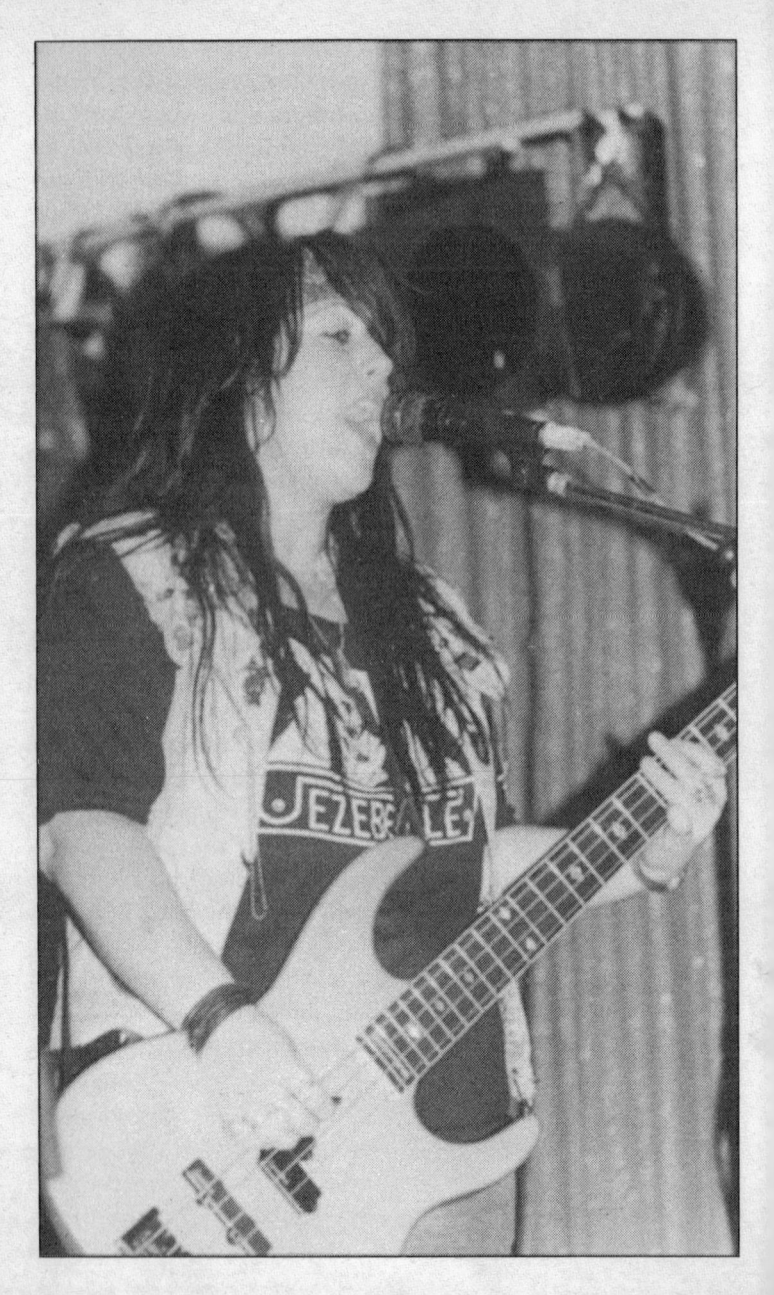

7
Sneha

MY CULTURE AFFECTS EVERY ASPECT OF MY LOOKS

Sneha, (not her real name) an Asian girl of eighteen living with her family near Birmingham, wrote me a long letter, but with the strict proviso that I didn't ring her at home or try to contact her at all. If I wrote, I mustn't make it clear from the envelope what the letter was about, or mention the title of the book on the outside. She was clearly terrified of her family discovering that she had written to me.

Her parents come originally from Mauritius, but Sneha was born in England. She feels that their culture is not her *culture, and they have had many arguments about the way she dresses; in particular a recent, violent one about wanting to cut her hair. She didn't want the fact that she had written to me to be discovered, and perhaps be seen by her parents as another act of disobedience, causing another row. At the moment she is going along with their wishes, wearing what they want her to and keeping her hair shoulder-length, but she feels extremely frustrated and isolated, and can't wait to leave home.*

'My family and I *always* argue over looks and clothes. I wanted to cut my hair short, and they allowed it for a while, until they discovered from a "friend" that I am a lesbian, and then they tried everything they could to stop me dressing as I used to. The last time I cut my hair my father beat me up very badly, and threw his weightlifting equipment at me. I decided then that I didn't want to be a martyr, and since then I haven't been near a hairdresser's.

I used to wear jeans and jackets and shirts but my parents burned them on the same day my dad beat me up, and after that

How Do I Look?

I had to wear saris. This restriction was lifted after a while, and now I can wear jeans again. My hair is now shoulder-length and will have to stay that way.

I suppose that my jeans, etc., were the traditional "butch" look, so that when my family learned of my lesbianism they saw my dress sense as one of the roots of this, and believed that by changing the way I looked, they could change the way I am. Since I can't dress the way I like, I try to go as far as I can whilst still making a feeble attempt at femininity. I wear jeans to university, as everyone else does. But I've become scruffier and scruffier, and although I do keep myself immaculately clean, I can't be bothered about my clothes any more. They get washed whenever I can be bothered, or whenever my mother raids my bedroom.

My culture – or rather, that of my parents – affects every aspect of my looks. Most young Asian or Asian-Mauritian girls have long hair; very few have short hair. Short hair is strictly forbidden for me not only because of my culture, but because of my lesbianism. This, incidentally, is viewed as a serious, punishable defect. If I was living in Mauritius, the time I could spend in jeans would be restricted, as young women seldom wear trousers; the Punjabi dress, with its tight-fitting trousers, is acceptable, though. As most of the older women wear saris, they consider fashionable clothes to be unnecessary and irrelevant, and can't understand the desires of someone like me, who wants to dress in a fashionable manner in the Western world. Shopping with my mother is a tedious experience, producing little or no results.

My mother is a jumble-sale dresser – that is, when she's not wearing a sari. She believes fashion to be a Western concept, and tells me that the only other clothes an Asian woman needs besides a sari is a "top" and a "nice skirt". But what she calls "nice", I call frumpy, and refuse to wear, and then the arguments start up again.

I think your mother has a big effect on your self-image, and I've learned nothing but bad habits from my own mother. She tells me I'm "fat" and is always making derogatory remarks and criticising. She is concerned about the size of the portions of food I eat. She herself eats very little, and she attempts to fit me into what she sees as her future role by teaching me to do the same. She is on a constant diet.

After I was born she put on a lot of weight, and although eventually she lost most of it, my birth was seen as to blame for her weight problem, and throughout my childhood she reminded me of this. As a teenager she had been frail and very light, and although now she is two stone heavier, and healthier for it, she still believes that young women should be thin, even skeletally so. This is a cultural belief as well as a personal one. It is easier for a husband to be found for a thin, and therefore supposedly beautiful, girl than for a plump one.

My mother taught me that the female body is something to be ashamed of. It must, at all costs, be covered up. She didn't just switch off the television during love scenes in a film, for instance, but even if a scantily clad woman was shown on a beach or something.

I had been told about periods at primary school when I was ten years old, but apart from that, the only information I had was what I got through talking to friends at school, because some had older sisters who had already started. I was twelve years old when I started my periods. I immediately knew what it was, but the thought of having to tell my mother terrified me. She'd never even mentioned them and I was sure she'd think I was unclean. When I did eventually tell her she was really embarrassed, and tried telling me that I was making it up! Then she said I'd cut myself. She refused to believe that anyone could start at that age; she'd been sixteen when hers had started. I was left feeling really dirty and confused, and I cried for a month.

By the time I was thirteen I already had a 36-inch bust, and during games lessons other girls would snigger, make remarks, and generally treat me like an abnormality. Any sport involving running was not only embarrassing, it was also extremely painful, because I never wore a proper fitting bra. Again, my mother refused to believe that I, at thirteen, could have the same size bust as her, and made me wear bras which were *much* too small

How Do I Look?

for me, causing the girls in the changing rooms at school to snigger even more.

Not surprisingly, nowadays I hate my breasts, and wish I didn't have them at all. If they were in proportion with the rest of my body, it would be better, then I wouldn't look top-heavy. To loads of people having heavy breasts means you are an "easy lay", or else it supposedly equals having no intelligence. If someone like Faith Brown wears a low-cut dress on television, her cleavage is all anyone looks at.

On the other hand, I think it would be great if television companies employed more large women (not just large-breasted women). Claire Rayner and Jeni Barnett are the only two I can think of at the moment. The rest are all Selina Scotts and Sue Lawleys. These are the only role models for young women; you feel inferior if you don't come up to those standards, even though you know it's a ridiculous stereotype. For instance, everyone makes such a fuss of Elizabeth Taylor when she loses weight, pampering her and commenting on how good she looks, but when she regains it, as she always does, we are told how ugly and inflated she is, and even *she* does not escape comparison – with Joan Collins. The fact is, Elizabeth Taylor is a plump woman who is exceptionally beautiful that way. She is simply the victim of the kind of prejudice which all plump women experience in their everyday lives, including me.

I constantly compare my body to other women's bodies, whether it's on television, or amongst my friends – I can't help myself. Most of my friends are thin, and sometimes I have this paranoiac feeling that they are using me. Beside me they look even slimmer, and I start thinking: maybe that's the only reason they are friends with me? I start wishing I looked like them, with elfin figures, no breasts and no hips. Whenever we're out together they won't go near a food shop, even if we're out for the whole day. I'm reluctant to say I'm hungry because I know the response will be: "That figures".

I am often secretive about what I eat, trying to hide it from my friends and family. My family think I should only eat at meal times, and only in small quantities, but I need more than that –

my stomach rumbles all the time between meals. My family can't understand why I might need to eat more, and tell me it's greediness. To avoid arguments I end up stealing food from the kitchen, or buying it elsewhere. I always eat well at university at lunch time, including a pudding, because I know that when I get home I will have to eat minute quantities. My mother doesn't cook very much food, and if I were to cook my own she would see it as greed and put a stop to it.

At home the pattern is always the same. My father and brothers eat first. My father sits in the living room in front of the television, my brothers in the dining room in silence. During this time my mother is in the kitchen washing up. Then I eat – in the dining room, alone – the boys having finished. My mother eats whatever is left in front of the television. The cultural rule is: men first.

I suppose I am plump – according to the "Height and Weight" charts I am on the heavy side of OK, but my weight has stayed the same since I was fourteen, so I know it's not true that I'm overeating, or greedy. Another of my friends – the only one who comes into this category – is as plump as I am, and when we go out together we eat as much as we want, whenever we want. When we are together there's no competition; neither of us feels better than or inferior to the other. In her company I feel she is my friend because she likes me, and not because she looks good beside me.

Boys do not have the same pressures as we do, they are not taught that image is so important; the media, society, and especially parents give them this impression. But they do have other pressures: to get a well-paid job, for instance. And if a boy is seen to be too concerned with his appearance, he gets called, amongst other things, a "poofter". So they are victims of pressures about looks, too, but in a different way.

What really angers me is the exploitation of young women like us by advertisers, to sell their products. Usually the girl shown is nothing to do with the product anyway; the Cadbury's Flake advert shows a pretty, pouting blonde woman wearing a slip. I can't see any connection between her and the product. The

How Do I Look?

other thing is, there are hardly any girls of Middle Eastern or Asian appearance in adverts or magazines. They are all white, mostly with blonde or light-brown hair. The advertisers obviously wish to give the idea that their products are for blondes or light-skinned people only, or maybe that if you use their product you will suddenly be transformed into a seductive beauty with a string of young men at your fingertips. Plump women are never featured either. In fact, the only time you see pictures of plump women are on the "before" and "after" photographs of the latest diet aid. Even clothes for "the larger woman" are usually modelled on women who are scarcely more than a size 12.

The women in adverts are always really feminine. This is stupid. Many, if not most, women are not glamorous and feminine – at least not most of the time. Women with hardly any make-up and short haircuts are never shown, as this would be the stereotypical lesbian, which advertisers are at pains to avoid! Since I am a short, plump, Asian young woman, with glasses and shortish hair, I've never found an advert with a woman looking anything like me.

I don't like the way I look, most of the time, for all the reasons I've just given. People think if you're small, you're there to be downtrodden, and they have a stack of prejudices about all the other things that I happen to be. Sometimes I think: if people don't like the way I look, that's their problem. Other times, I feel so repressed and pressurised, I long to change the way I look, to be taller and lose some weight, but I know that's not the answer.'

III
Conflicts

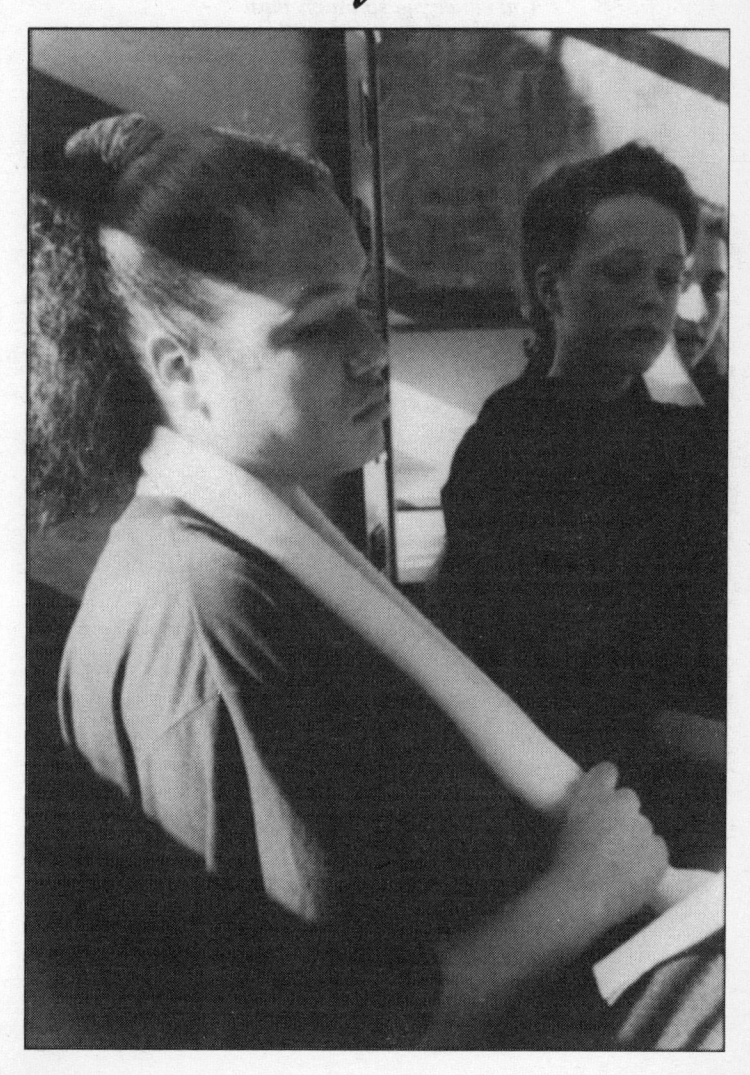

A LONG OVERDUE POEM TO MY EYES

Poor brown slit eyes
You cause me so much pain
But for you, I would be,
Totally invisible.

When young,
You filled with tears
At the slightest provocation.
When children teased,
It was because of you
They hated me.

In story books,
Her big blue eyes opened wide.
But you, you narrowed into slits.

Hard brown slit eyes
Echoes of the pain
You mirror back the world,
And I can see them all,
Drowning there.

Soft brown slit eyes
Windows of the Soul
I can see you staring back
Frank, open, lovely.

Meiling Jin

We may feel that we are being neurotic if we have a bad self-image, vain if we have a good one, or trivial to care at all. Trivial or shallow, in particular, are criticisms levelled at young women for their concern over their appearance; one of the worst current insults you can throw at an actress or pop star is that she's a bimbo – concerned only with her looks and nothing else. There doesn't seem to be any equivalent insult for a boy. It is also assumed that a bimbo is unintelligent, couldn't possibly have an interest in anything other than clothes and make-up. So to be concerned with fashion, to dress up and have fun with clothes, is to be stupid, even whilst every single day the fashion, advertising, and plastic surgery businesses (not to mention slimming aids, diet books, fitness centres, cosmetics industry) pump millions of pounds into all these things.

It is obvious that image *is* important, both to the young woman concerned with her self-image and to those involved in promoting a certain kind of image, a certain look. Sometimes a girl is in conflict with her culture or religion in how she wants to dress and express herself, as Sneha (Chapter 7) describes; sometimes a young woman enjoys dressing a certain way but discovers that there are prejudices and stereotypes about the way she wants to look; conflicts that might come from within, or from her family, her job, or the outside world.

8
Helen

I CAN'T HELP BLAME THE WAY I LOOK

Helen is twenty-three, and lives on her own in a student flat in Leicester. She wrote a long and moving letter, describing her terrifying experience of being raped whilst on holiday with two friends. Clearly Helen has looked for 'explanations' to help her deal with such a painful experience, and the one she seems to have come up with is that she was picked on for the way she looks. It is easy to see why a girl might come to this conclusion. We've all seen pictures of Page 3 girls and pornographic images of women showing the female body in a constantly inviting, sexual way (just walking into a newsagent's on a Sunday morning often means you are surrounded by them) and it is hardly surprising if girls themselves, as well as men, sometimes feel confused; believing that girls might 'want' to be raped, or are asking for trouble, if they dress up to go out, or behave independently by going out or walking home alone.

Although Helen is aware that her feelings of being to blame are irrational and unjustified, sadly, they are not easy to rid herself of. Many girls spoke to me of how a fear of being raped or 'hassled' affected the way they dressed and how they felt about their looks and bodies.

'I suppose there are other girls who have had the same experience as me, and that my talking about it in this book might help them feel less isolated. It is very hard to describe what happened to me, but here goes:

Several years ago, I went on holiday with some friends. Within a couple of days they had paired off with English boys whom they met in the Spanish bars. I suppose I was surprised, maybe even a bit shocked, as I had assumed we would be spending the holiday together, laughing and drinking. I really did feel very left out, and left out of something important, a feeling I'd had before. They both had boyfriends in England, I didn't. They wore pastel pink sundresses, and I wore dark clothes and had spiky hair. They did pressure me quite a lot about how I looked, but I never gave in to their attempts to convert me to pink; I wanted to look different, and in the main I was quite happy with my image.

On the third evening, I was sitting drinking alone and started talking to a man who offered to walk me back to the hotel. As he pointed out, it wasn't safe for me to go back on my own. I was flattered by his concern, and charmed by him. We left the bar together; one of my friends saw us leave and winked at us.

My memory gets very vague here. It's like bits of a film – I have only fragments, each image a few seconds long. I know that he kicked and punched me; I know he told me this was what I wanted, that no one would ever love me, and this was all I was fit for; and I know he raped me. I remember a sensation like a slug or a snake, something vile entering me, and I remember vomiting. I can hear myself running through a subway, sobbing and stumbling, with footsteps behind me, like a terrifying nightmare. It certainly was my worst nightmare, and I don't think I will ever get over it.

I didn't tell anyone for ages. I thought he had been right, and that what happened to me on that oily beach was all I was fit for. For a while I was scared that I was pregnant; I had a disgusting sense of something alien inside me, like maggots or a cancer. I think that was more to do with how I felt about what had happened than a real fear of pregnancy. In any case – thank God – eventually my period came and I knew I wasn't pregnant. But I blamed my body for what had happened, I hated it, I hated having breasts, I thought my body was saying: Hey, here I am, come and get me! and I was terrified whenever I walked down the street. From that time on, it seemed as though I loathed myself and looked for ways to punish my body.

It is still so difficult to talk about rape, or having been raped.

How Do I Look?

I feel that because I can't bring myself to talk about it, but on the other hand I can't forget it, I joke instead about hating my body, or hating being a girl, or hating men, then I get drunk and cry. People describe me as "hysterical"; this only makes me feel worse. Sometimes I go out and pick up strange men in clubs because that seems to fit the self-image that I've adopted – I don't know if that makes sense. But in the long run it only makes me feel worse about myself.

I don't know if I could ever have a relationship, the way I feel about my body. I've never even managed to get through a job interview, even if it's a woman doing the interviewing; I just have this feeling that she is looking at me and judging me for all the wrong reasons. Sitting in a small room with a strange man asking me questions is pure hell.

Although I'm starting to cope with the idea that the rape wasn't my fault, I can't get rid of the feeling that something about my appearance singled me out. I think that because I was wearing dark clothes and not giggling, he saw me as a challenge. I have a feeling now, as if I'm walking around with a sign on my back saying "Kick me", or "I'm a prat", the sort of horrible joke kids play on each other, because I feel as though that's exactly how people treat me.

Before the rape, I don't think I felt that bad about myself. My parents are very accepting; my mum encourages me to dress for comfort rather than fashion. Photos of my mum taken twenty-five years ago could be of me, we look so alike – but she does think I'm too scruffy. My parents were quite honest with me about things to do with sex, periods, etc. I had a very scientific explanation about periods from my mum, with a warning not to tell my father or younger sister that I'd started.

It's not that I'm particularly unhappy with the shape of my body or with my image, it's just that I worry all the time about what people think about me, what impression they are getting. When I think of what the "ideal" look is for a girl, I always imagine it as someone looking happy, and that is the one thing I know I *don't* look.

I'm not sure what I'm aiming for when I look in the mirror.

Conflicts

Some days I'm happy with the way I look, others I'm not. I don't know if this is to do with my lipstick or my attitude. The sad part is that I've come to hate my body so much, I blame it for everything, and now I can't let anyone get close to me, to reassure me.'

9
Louisa
WHY CAN'T I WEAR WHAT I LIKE?

You don't have to have experienced rape or sexual attack to feel that your life is affected by the fear of it. Louisa is twenty and from Yorkshire. Outgoing and engaging, she is the only girl in a household of brothers and confessed to being the pet of the family. She is about to leave home to go to drama school. She met me in London wearing a wide-brimmed hat, khaki shorts and a loose white top; she says she loves showing off, feels her legs are her best feature and that short skirts suit her. But having fun dressing up to 'show off' sometimes makes her anxious that people are getting the wrong idea, misinterpreting her look. She knows that wanting to look good, or sexy, doesn't mean she's 'asking for it', but that belief was shaken by a recent incident, and by the overprotective reaction of her brother to her when she told him about it.

'A few nights ago I went round to my boyfriend's house. It's this really creepy area, a dead-end road in a red-light district, and when I got there I discovered I didn't have my key and he wasn't in, so I was locked out. The only thing I could do was sit outside his house on the doorstep. It was early evening, about seven o'clock; I was wearing a short skirt and no coat, because the weather was warm, and we were supposed to be going out. But pretty quickly I started to get all this hassle: these guys coming up to me, driving past in cars and stopping, calling out things to me. I was beginning to feel really nervous.

Then this one guy stopped and parked his car just across the road. He was watching me. I was terrified, I tried not to look at him, I tried pulling my skirt down over my knees. Then he got out of the car and said something to me. I told him I was waiting for my boyfriend, and he got back in his car but still sat there, looking at me.

It was horrible. I was terrified, I sat there until my boyfriend came back, I didn't even have enough money for my bus fare or to make a phone call to my brother and ask him to come and pick me up. I felt so cross with myself, so stupid for wearing a short skirt. But on the other hand, I was furious; I thought: this is ridiculous, why shouldn't I go out wearing what I want without getting hassle?

When I told my big brother about the whole thing, he said I was bloody stupid; I only had myself to blame. "If you ever ring me and you're out on your own and it's after ten o'clock, I'm not coming to pick you up" – that's what he told me. I look up to my brother, what he says goes with me, so that really hurt. The thing is, he says he knows a lot about the world, he knows what men are like, he says he's just worried for me. But when he said that, I felt to blame for the situation I was in. I didn't wear a short skirt for ages after that.

I feel very strong most of the time; I'm big and tall and I could outrun most people. I don't very often feel frightened, but then I don't often put myself in that vulnerable position. In the summer men can wear shorts or whatever they like (and sometimes they look revolting in them, too!) and no one says anything to them about it. I think most men are under the impression that we all want to look like Samantha Fox, but if you have a big chest it's very difficult to handle all the hassle you get when you walk down the street.

If I was walking past a building site, I'd put my head down, trying not to have eye contact with anyone, but I'd be expecting it anyway – not because I'm pretty, but because if it's summer and you're a girl and, say, wearing shorts, it's inevitable. When I got past I'd put my head up again, as if to say, "I don't care". I wouldn't be embarrassed so much as angry. I'd feel like saying, "Have you had your eyeful, then?" I've said that before to men: "Have you had a long enough look?"

I used to be flattered when I was about thirteen. I can

remember the very first time it happened – I was out walking the dog with my mum and a car tooted at us, and my mum said, "Oh, someone thinks your bottom's nice". And I thought: Don't be silly, it isn't me. Then not long after, we were both walking under some scaffolding – she was already under it and out of view – when a workman whistled, so I knew it was for me, not her. I thought: Wow, somebody's noticed me! Someone thinks I'm pretty! I quickly realised that that's not the case at all, they do it to everybody. You're a girl, they're blokes, they seem to think it's their duty to comment; it doesn't matter what you're wearing.

If you wear short skirts with opaque tights and clumpy shoes, that's a slightly different look. People know what that means, and you get less hassle. But if you wear light tights – you know, sheer tights and a short skirt and high heels – people seem to think that means you're dressed up, a different type. And having my kind of build, being quite big and wearing miniskirts, I know that sometimes it gets me the wrong kind of attention from boys only interested in physical relationships. Tons of people have said to me, "Oh, it's nice to have a rounded body", but personally I'm not very happy with the body I've got.

When I was eighteen, about six months before my A levels, I stopped eating for about three months, then every now and then, about every week, I'd binge really heavily. Afterwards I would feel so guilty that I tried to make myself sick but actually, it never worked. Then I felt even more depressed. One day my mum sat me on the bed and started talking to me. She said there must be more to it than just worrying about wanting a small waist, and she was right: out it came. It was a lot to do with the school I was at, and worrying about these other girls being prettier or cleverer than me. I didn't have a boyfriend, and I was convinced that it was because I was too fat. Since then, whenever I have any worries, I've focused on my weight. I know that's the only thing in my life that I can change and attack. Like – I know these girls who sleep with their boyfriends to get taken out, and I know that my body could be a kind of power as well, I could get what I want with it. All the time I'm either bingeing (in secret) or doing loads of exercise; I really feel desperate to lose weight because I'm going to be a bridesmaid soon, and I don't want to look like a splodge at my brother's wedding. I know I'm damaging my body and health, but I don't know how to stop.'

Louisa's confusion about sex, and whether her body is 'a kind of power' or a vulnerability, leaving her open to sexual attack, has turned into an obsession with losing weight, and wishing to lose the breasts and curviness that cause so many problems in her life. The connection between girls suffering from eating disorders and violently hating their own bodies, and sexual violence in society, struck me more and more powerfully as I listened to girls talking about periods, body shape and size, and how they feel about their bodies.

Recent research has shown up a link between girls who have suffered from some (often seemingly unimportant or minor) kind of sexual abuse and those who later go on to develop eating problems. Many girls wrote to me of exactly this kind of thing – for instance, Amelia, aged thirteen:

> There was this boy at school. He kept touching me up, touching my breasts. It ended in a fight – I hit him, he hit me – then the teacher came in and broke the whole thing up. Now I feel so embarrassed and wish I didn't have breasts at all, or I try to hide them with baggy T-shirts. I'm glad that since I lost weight, they're hardly noticeable.

Many girls longed to 'lose' their bottoms or breasts or stomachs – and not just those with eating disorders. Many girls were saying to me, 'I can't cope with having breasts, the hassle it brings, the fear of rape or the jokes and remarks from boys, the idea that I must be a slag or a "goer", so rather than try to deal with the whole world (which I can't), I'll just turn all my anger inwards against myself, against the thing I can control: my body.'

How Do I Look?

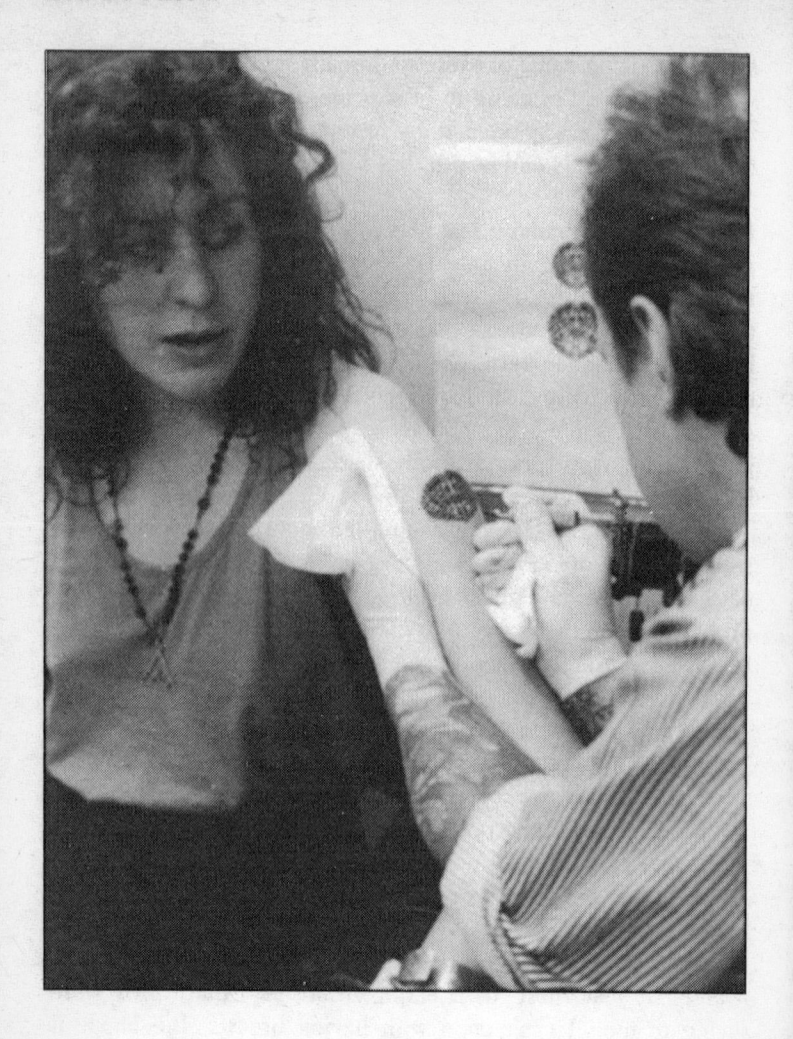

10
Ann

WHO WANTS TO BE DRESSED BY THEIR MUM AT EIGHTEEN?

Ann opened the door of the large student house in South London where she lives, wearing a cotton print dress in deep colours, and my first impression was of someone fair and small and limping. It was possible to think, as she herself points out, that she had merely tripped over a plug or something; in fact Ann has an artificial leg. When she was fourteen she developed bone cancer and the doctors advised amputation of one leg. The loss of her leg was a devastating experience; apart from the practical side of coping with hair loss due to the chemotherapy (radiation treatment for cancer) and the difficulties of learning to walk with her artificial leg, Ann's self-image underwent an enormous change.

She describes herself as 'big and strong', even though she readily admits she probably isn't actually that big – that's just the way she feels about herself, the way she feels she has to be. Now twenty-four, she came to London orginally from Gloucestershire, and has only just moved 'south of the river' to start a new job. The house we sat in was still in chaos, so she led me to the sunny kitchen, where we talked and drank coffee, surrounded by boxes and plants and the smell of paint.

'At fourteen I thought of myself as having potential – the usual things: getting a boyfriend, going out with my friends – then after the loss of my leg, all that was shattered. My image of myself altered radically. I didn't go back to school after coming out of hospital, I felt that all that potential had gone; I just stayed at home watching "Rainbow" and "Play School". I thought: No one is going to find me attractive, because I've got one leg, so I might as well forget it. I saw myself as a write-off as far as boyfriends were concerned.

The chemotherapy made my hair fall out, I was really bald. My mum used to pick my hair off the pillow while I was asleep so that I wouldn't see how much I was losing, and at that time I was too ill to get up and go and look in the mirror. When I did eventually look in the mirror my hair was in patches, like little bits of baby hair. They wanted me to wear this wig, a gross, thick, nylon thing like something out of the Nolan sisters. It was hideous.

I refused to wear it. Sometimes I'd wear a headscarf, but mainly I just didn't go out. Anyway, I felt too ill. Once they stopped the drugs they were giving me, my hair started to come back. But I wouldn't have my photograph taken at that time at all. My family kept trying to make me, to make me feel OK about myself. But I felt dreadful, like a bloated lump with one leg and no hair, so there aren't any photos of me at that time at all. I never had any taken until I felt happy with myself. Now I'm happy to be photographed.

This was in the heady days of 1978, when I first lost my leg, when very flared trousers were in. Platforms were out, high heels were in, but also flat shoes, those nurse's shoes with laces, and circular skirts and long flared coats. Also big trousers with big tops – it was all coming to an end, but it was still OK to wear them. It was brilliant from the point of view of having one leg, because everything was hidden. I never wore skirts. I never wore anything that hugged my body. In those days the artificial leg you were given didn't meet the skin; you had to wear thick woollen socks over the join where the artificial leg met your own leg, and a metal belt to hold it in place, which pulled your body over to one side. My body was deformed by the weight of the belt to hold the leg in place. Obviously I couldn't wear tops that were short which would show where the belt was, so that summer was terrible. I wore horrible hippy flared dresses, which I hated.

I didn't know anyone else or any girls my age with my disability. If I had known someone who looked similar to me, we

Conflicts

could have walked down the street together, wearing similar clothes or something; we'd be holding each other's hands in a sense, it would have been easier. As if we were saying: Sod you, I don't care.

Everyone likes to hang around with people with a similar image, it gives you more confidence to experiment. By the time I went to college, I did feel more confident. I dyed my hair every colour under the sun, and I was in this all-women band, we wore lots and lots of make-up and these really baggy dresses in wild colours, which covered our whole bodies – we all dressed the same. I didn't think anyone was aware of my leg; I do limp, but for all they knew I might have just tripped over a plug or something. Then one day, I was in this car with some blokes, and one of them said, "Have you heard about this band, with a really good one-legged woman bass player?" I was just cracking up; they didn't realise it was me! In the end I told them, and they shut up. I think that's how you learn people's true reactions to you, but by that time I was starting to feel better about myself, and I could laugh at them.

People think the word "one-legged" is funny. In fact, people think being hard of hearing is funny, or being short-sighted. When that word applies to you, obviously your image of yourself suffers as you try to separate who you are from what people think you are. I mean, Kylie Minogue in a wheelchair would not be Kylie Minogue, because if she went on "Top of the Pops" it would be: "Here's tragic Kylie, here's a scene from her hospital bed", then she'd sink into never-never land – bye-bye.

The feeling of being "disabled" – I feel that more when I'm forced into situations where I can't be myself. Say at work, I can wear what I want. I'd never accept a job where I had to wear a skirt. Wearing a skirt and high heels – that makes me feel *so* disabled, and unattractive. Nowadays, in artificial leg technology, you can get this special foot where you put an Allen key in the heel and hey presto: you can wear high heels. But this is horrible, because walking with an artificial leg makes you wobbly anyway, without the added problem of high heels. There are also these artificial plastic toes that you fit over your artificial foot, so you can wear open-toed sandals. Imagine that!

Shoes, now, aren't a problem. I have a whole wide range: black suede pumps, black boots with low heels – I have to have a pretty low heel. That's fine, because there are lots of shoes in the shops with low heels to choose from. I wear DMs like everybody else. I wouldn't want to wear high heels anyway. I never even look at them in shops. I think they're old-fashioned, for older women, or women who work in the city, not for girls.

I mostly wear jeans and trousers and leggings, not skirts. I wore this dress to work today, because we had a meeting, but mostly I wear what I want. Not that it's that easy to shop for clothes, that's why most disabled girls end up wearing what people have given them. Or they're dressed by their mothers. But who wants their mum to dress them when they're eighteen! Or undress them, for that matter.

If you're a young disabled girl – say, in a wheelchair – it's sheer culture shock to put yourself somewhere like Oxford Circus. You can't get down the escalator, everyone's looking at you, then there are all these other young things flipping around the changing rooms in the shops. I never go in changing rooms, because I'm not prepared for people to say, "Oh, look at her leg!" I usually take something off the peg, hope that it fits, take it home and if it doesn't, try taking it back.

All able-bodied people go on about how horrible the changing-room experience is – how awful because my bra is dirty, or I'm too fat or too thin – but disabled girls: how do you even begin to assess your own emotions on entering a changing room with young able-bodied women, most of them slim but all saying, "Oh, I've got a horrible body", when you're in a wheelchair, just wanting to try on a pair of trousers?

I do feel self-conscious in some situations. I mean, I can swim or cycle, but I can't go to aerobics or do those kind of things, because I'd feel too self-conscious. When I go swimming, there is a lot to think about: I have to work out whether my artificial leg will fit in the locker, then the problem of how to get into the water, and I *know* people will be staring at me. When I go abroad on holiday, I think: I'm here for two weeks, I can either sit here fully dressed for a whole fortnight, or I can take my leg off and jump in the pool. I know some people will look, but eventually they'll get used to it; say, "Oh, that's the girl with one leg", and nothing more. It's worth it because it's lovely when you're in the water, you're of equal status with everyone else, it's nice to have the movement, to float around, unrestrained.

Parties are another situation where I know I'll probably feel self-conscious. When I'm getting ready for a party – you know, you have a bath some time in the early afternoon or evening, you work out what to wear, you lay the things out on the bed that you vaguely know you look nice in, you roughly know what make-up suits you . . . well, that's the point when I start thinking about my leg, and whether it will show. I'm thinking: I'm not wearing this, or I'm not wearing that, my leg shows in that; but it's funny, it's only really at parties that I worry about things like that. About clothes clinging. I suppose parties are where you feel most aware of sex, and it is a problem sometimes, trying to feel sexy, when you are what most people consider "unsexy", by only having one leg.

But despite how I felt at first about myself when I lost my leg, I haven't really had that many problems with boyfriends. In a way, it's ended up being a good test to measure potentially good relationships against bad ones, because say I went out with someone and at a party they said, "Sit on me lap, darling", and then they said, "Oh God, you've only got one leg" – well, I'd know they wouldn't be worth going out with!

I met this bloke in August who said, "I'll only consider going out with you if you lose three stone". I was flabbergasted, it was absolutely against all my politics, but I thought: just to show you, I will. I did easily lose a stone and a half, but then I thought: I don't want him anyway. I think he caught me at a vulnerable moment, when I was more worried about myself than I am now.

When I was younger, I thought: people will see me coming, and only see a leg, then later they'll see the person. You think at first that you have no choice, that it's not up to you to decide on things like boyfriends – he's sexy or he's ugly – that you can just forget it. Now I have my own friends and we never really talk about it. I'd say I was happy with the way I look 90 per cent of the time; I can't imagine myself any other way.'

IV
Obsessions

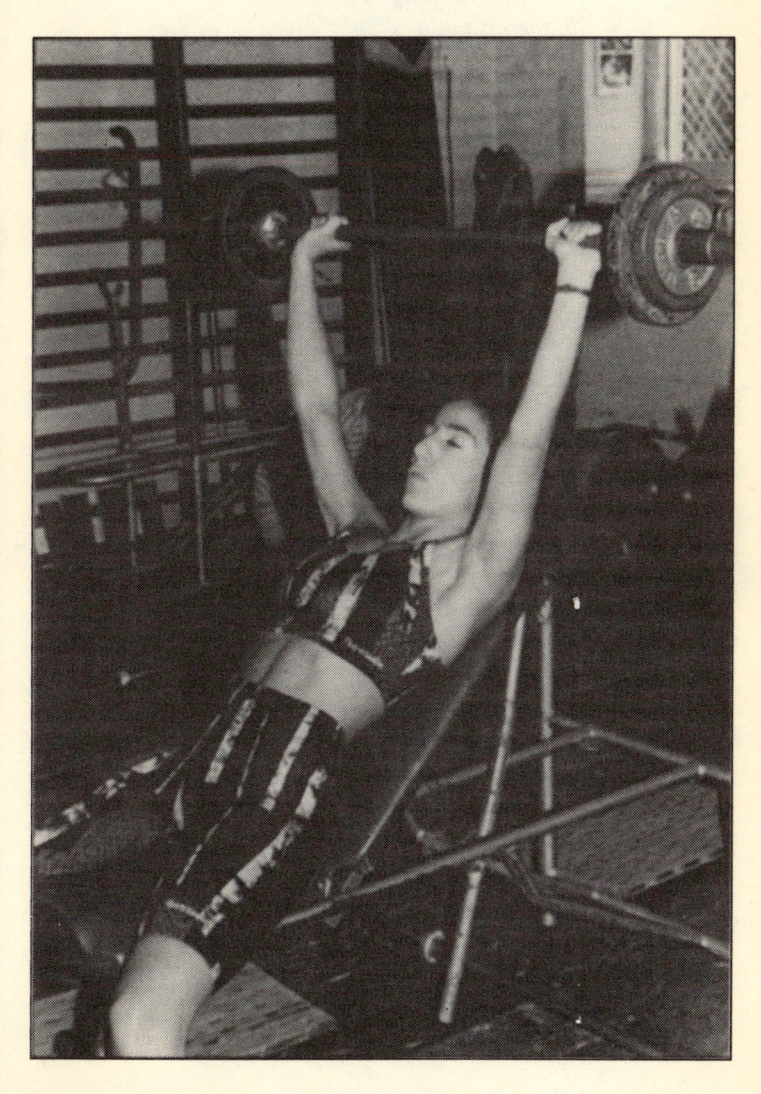

ANOREXIA

*Only occasionally
do the crumbly ribs
frighten with their frailty.
Only occasionally
and quickly forgotten
from the cocoon beneath the sheets,
where hugged thigh flesh
demands endless black coffee
and banishes the chip.*

*Very occasionally
my heart swells
at the rounded figure
of the 8 inside my jeans.
But my hand on jutting hip
reminds: the jut is not enough
and come Weigh Day
(the Sabbath)
the sacred scales proffer no absolution:
'Seven pounds still to lose
And to lose . . .'*

Anon

Anorexia, where self-image and reality can be so at odds that a girl can look in the mirror and see someone hugely fat when in fact she is skeletal, is growing amongst teenage girls, and beginning to affect more Black and Asian girls living in Britain. It is even increasing amongst boys. The media dub it the 'slimming disease', and shake their heads in dismay at foolish girls (and now boys) who 'suffer from' this 'bewildering' 'illness'. Compulsive eating, on the other hand, receives less sympathy and rather more tut-tutting and remarks of the 'should have more self-discipline' variety. But both are only extremes of something that is considered perfectly normal: that girls and young women should want to change themselves. Paula Yates, for instance, admits in an interview in *Woman* magazine that she is so thin that she had to put on weight before she could become pregnant. Once she'd had the baby, she immediately set about getting back to her 'normal' weight, even though that weight was so low that her body could not function normally. Yet she isn't considered anorexic, she is simply considered (by some) attractive.

In researching this book I read a quote from a well-known doctor working with girls with eating disorders: he said that in the West, if you are female and do not have hang-ups about your body, you are abnormal. In one shape or size this was said to me often in writing this book, and always by women and girls themselves. I know what they mean, but I disagree. I read articles in women's magazines that began: 'We all need to cut down every now and then', or 'We all hate something about ourselves, whether it's our stomach or our nose' . . . but do we? And why should we? What's wrong with us the way we are?

In the following chapters, two young women describe this longing to change – to change their bodies and, they imagined, themselves – and how these longings turned into obsessions.

11
Alison

WITHOUT MY EXERCISE I'M A CRYING WRECK

Alison is eighteen and has, as she puts it in her long letter, 'never reached adolescence'. She has never had a period; at eleven she was diagnosed as anorexic and hospitalised for ten weeks. When she was realeased she had gained some weight, but it was fear of rehospitalisation rather than a true recovery that kept her from losing all the weight again. Her obsession has taken the form of compulsive exercising: huge amounts of daily exercise, without which she feels panic-stricken and lost.

Alison's story is extreme, but many of the things she says will strike a chord with other girls. In particular, her hatred of her body and her description of her breasts as 'useless lumps of flesh' echo the feelings of other girls I spoke to about the female body. Pornography and a fear of rape play a huge part in girls' mistrust of their own bodies. Helen and Louisa talk about this in Chapters 8 and 9.

It was striking that many of the girls I spoke to with anorexia or bulimia (an eating disorder similar to anorexia, but in which sufferers make themselves sick or take laxatives to keep their weight down; both methods are extremely dangerous to health) told of an incident (which they often insist was small or insignificant) of sexual harassment or abuse which marked the start of their body obsession. Often they had not told anyone about what they saw as a trivial event, but had buried their feelings of embarrassment and fear until they resurfaced in the shape of an obsession.

Although you may feel that Page 3 models, pornographic magazines, videos and films have no relevance to your life, and certainly no relevance to your obsession with losing weight or remaining slim, it is easy to see how such images of womanhood can contribute to a sense of vulnerability to rape, or just confusion over whether having breasts and thighs means you are always sexually available. And I do not think that Helen is unusual or unfathomable in translating this into a hatred of her own body, a fear of its femininity, unpredictability and curviness, and a longing to keep it all 'under control'.

Alison's account makes very clear her terror of periods and of having a woman's body, of becoming a woman. Although there are many complex factors in anorexia, I have chosen to concentrate on this sense of self-hatred and dissatisfaction with her body and image; on those areas which are directly about the question: 'How do I look?'

'"Jogged round reservoir (4 miles) in snow. Slippery again. Swam at Mosley Road (50 lengths) . . . had a 10-mile cycle, lunch, exercises . . ." This is a quote from my diary in December 1986, when I was fourteen. Before I was hospitalised I would walk at breakneck pace for several hours each day, trying to convince myself and others that I was enjoying it. I even walked to the hospital, rather than travelling in the car with my desperate parents, for the psychiatrist's appointment which resulted in my ten-week enforced stay.

When I was released, I was so relieved that I swore I would lead a normal life – no more endless walks. I would only start up ballet again "for pleasure". But within days meal times became battlegrounds between my family and me, and I needed the long walks more than ever, to let off steam. I kept starting new regimes, then finding I couldn't give them up. Without my exercise, I was a crying wreck. I would go out in all weathers, at all times: exercise was an addiction. I took up dancing again with a vengeance; grinding through as many as six lessons a week. I cursed myself for lack of balance; I was determined to be a professional dancer. Everyone, including me, was convinced that I loved dancing. But it was hatred of myself that drove me, not love of dancing.

Exercise, measuring food and then eating it, dominated my

How Do I Look?

life. I had no time for friends, relaxation or pleasure. But one day a girl at school invited me to her home, and we began to see more of each other, became friends. That was the first occasion when I saw my exercising as an irritating use of time, because it got in the way of our friendship. I also began to describe my obsessions to my friend, who was wonderfully tolerant, and I became aware, in telling her, how ridiculous my routines were. The amounts of exercise I did meant that I had to eat more than my father! For years I convinced myself that I hated eating, and loved the dance lessons. My new friend was the first step in questioning whether that was true.

It seems I have always been obsessed with the way I look. My parents kept a baby book about me until I was sixteen, and when I was three and a half they wrote: "Takes a great interest in her clothes and chooses her own outfit each morning. Makes some very original and attractive colour combinations. Loves long socks and prefers to keep shoes on and arms covered up. If weather is very hot . . . loves to take off all clothes and play with hose." When I was four years old the book reads: "Very fond of dressing up, especially in an old nylon nightdress – 'the princess dress'."

I remember this dress well. There are other entries describing my passion for clothes, and also my concern to look good – for example, it notes that I insisted on having long hair, despite problems of manageability. I remember terrible arguments when shopping for shoes – I wanted to have fashion shoes (high heels, pointed toes) like my friends, but Mum always made me have sensible shoes. Once, I was going to be a bridesmaid in a blue dress, and when I needed new shoes before the wedding, I refused to have blue shoes, insisting on brown ones. I used to click around in my mum's high-heeled shoes, and I especially loved her boots! I can remember a party dress that I loved – a white one with bright, tiny flowers on and lace trimming. It was so special, and I would have special party shoes which were gold or silver. Getting ready for a party at five years old was brilliant fun. At six and a half I loved making up my face, and at ten, the baby book recorded, I wanted to be a dress designer.

I never actually reached puberty, in terms of periods, although I can remember feeling lumps developing in my breasts, and being momentarily shocked before realising that I was growing up. My baby book says: "Slight breast development" at ten and a half years old. I went off to school camp for a few days when I was ten, and Mum suggested I took some sanitary towels with me in case my period started, but I dismissed this as silly and unnecessary. Also at ten and a half the baby book comments: "Is prudish about bodies". My father writes: "Is teased at school about being vain, and no wonder. Shows no interest in intellectual things. Prefers women's magazines to anything serious. Makes charts of calories in various foods and tries to make herself thinner, although she is quite slim."

From as young as ten I was very conscious of having fat thighs. I don't know exactly where this came from, or even whether or not they really were fat. I started buying exercise and diet books. The last entry in the baby book before I was hospitalised with anorexia reads: "Failed 11-plus exam. Took this disappointment very well." I stopped eating on my return from the summer camp mentioned earlier.

I still don't know which specific events led to my becoming anorexic. I don't think I am fully recovered, and today I am no taller or heavier than I was when I was released from hospital in 1983.

The hospital treatment consisted of a high-calorie diet, complete bed-rest for eight weeks, and chlorpromazine drugs. I was allowed to see my parents only three times a week. I saw a psychiatrist often during my stay, up to once a day, although the sessions seemed more like informal chats. I was weighed once a week, but never told my weight. This, as you can imagine, was a terrifying experience, and memories of my hospital stay still frighten me.

Today, I supose I don't exactly dislike my body, but neither do I like it much. My years of dancing, beginning long before I was anorexic, have made me very body-conscious, both in how my body looks and how it feels. I am unable to cope with the idea of being any heavier than I am now, and would not like to

How Do I Look?

have a period, since I would feel I had "let up" control over my body. I want to remain exceptionally thin, because then I am never likely to get fat. I realise that this must sound silly, but I don't know how to change it. I run three miles, or swim 40–60 lengths, six days a week, and also do an hour's stretching and strengthening exercises every day, which makes me quite fit, a feeling I enjoy. The stupid part is, recently I noticed a girl at our local swimming pool, painfully emaciated, like something out of a concentration camp, who came every morning to swim lengths, as I do. I plucked up the courage to talk to her, and felt this urgent need to tell her that she would eventually kill herself. I was desperate on her behalf, but on my own . . . I don't know why, but I can't see things that clearly. I know what I'm doing, I know it's self-destructive and dangerous, but because I'm not quite as terrifyingly thin as she was, I'm able to convince myself that I'm in control, and continue with my exercising mania.

I suppose I am happy being so "tiny"; it means I am able to surprise people with what is generally seen as my confident and outgoing personality.

I would find it very difficult to go into a situation, like a communal changing room in a big store, where other women would see my body. If I had to undress in front of them, I'd be wondering what they were thinking about my body – "Do they think I'm anorexic, or just plain thin? Do they think I'm crazy too?" I would be painfully aware of myself, convinced they were looking at me, and trying to act normally, without any idea what "normal" is. I'd be concerned as to whether I was wearing more layers of clothing than the other women, and whether anyone had noticed.

I do look at other women's bodies; I tell myself it's good for me to know what "ordinary" bodies look like. I always pity the average and fat ones, congratulating myself on having avoided such a flabby fate. I ask myself if I want to be more like the slim women whom I admire than like my own thin body. But usually I decide it's OK for them, but not for me – I couldn't bear it, I'd feel fat.

Although I know that the amount of exercise I do will keep

me fit, these days I feel guilty about doing "so little" exercise. I have a nagging sense of being unsatisfied with my behaviour, as though I was doing something morally wrong. I agree with eating disorder's therapist Marilyn Lawrence that "when complusive exercisers talk about how good their regime makes them feel, they are actually talking about wanting to be a good person. And you can't achieve that through exercise."

Proof of being a good person seems to me to be when other people show that they like, love or respect you. I have been convinced for a long time that people could not love, accept or respect me for the person I am, only for the amazing amount of exercise I can do.

I think that an exercise obsession is a symptom of lack of self-esteem and identity. I would tell other girls who suspect they have an exercise problem similar to mine to ask themselves the following questions: Do I take more exercise than is necessary for health and fitness? Do I really enjoy all my exercise? Why do I take as much exercise as I do? What do I want from exercise? What would happen if I took less exercise? Aren't there more important things in my life that I could spend the time on that is currently taken up with exercise?'

The above account was written to me in a long, beautifully typed letter. In some ways Alison seems very cool about her condition and has remained detached from the experiences she is describing. It is quite breathtaking, for instance, that her sympathies are so strong for another girl whom she sees as literally killing herself with exercise, yet she doesn't really extend her sympathies or concern towards herself.

Reading her account of her childhood, we are told of her early passion for clothes and looking good. But what she also inadvertently tells us is how much emphasis her parents (and all parents) tend to put on little girls looking good – providing dancing lessons, special party dresses, and constant compliments for being pretty. I think the fact that her parents kept a baby book on her until she was sixteen reveals the way in which a certain obsession was shown on *their* part with how she looks, and with her developing body.

And Alison's parents are not unusual. Most little girls are given toys which include dolls, make-up sets, and dressing-up outfits. Most of us were encouraged at one time to 'dress up' and look pretty. It seems cruel that what is encouraged and praised in girls as children (and is also, after all, an expression of identity and creativity which little boys too could benefit from) is suddenly, at age eleven seen as vanity, and a sign of low intellect.

Alison's baby book starts at three and a half. I have noticed since having a baby myself (a little boy) how attitudes about such things as 'prettiness' and looks start much younger than that. From the day they are born, girl babies and boy babies are 'labelled' in hospital, given a pink or blue tag, and then doctors, visitors and friends respond accordingly; remarking what 'strong' lungs he has if he's a boy, and what a 'dainty little thing' she is if she's a girl. Perhaps we could all be a lot more tolerant of ourselves for sometimes longing to be beautiful if we considered for how many years of our lives this had been held out to us as an ideal.

The baby book gives us another glimpse into parents' and societies' attitudes towards girls' bodies with the comment that Alison is 'prudish' about her body at ten, and the noting of her 'slight breast development'. Surely 'prudish' is simply a natural desire for privacy and separation which is an essential part of growing up; and surely having your parents writing about your breast development in a baby book is not very likely to make you feel unselfconscious about it!

I think that privacy and a sense of owning your own body and knowing its boundaries is quite a difficult thing for girls to achieve in a world in which female bodies are plastered on every billboard, and when you walk down the street those boundaries can so easily be invaded by men commenting on the size of your breasts or on what you are wearing. But developing a sense of this is essential to wellbeing; assertiveness training and learning self-defence can both help.

It is obvious that Alison has not recovered in any sense, and is

Obsessions

just managing to keep out of hospital by maintaining her weight at a low but not life-threatening level. Many girls said to me that you never recover from anorexia or bulimia or compulsive eating, but having suffered from all three for over seven years, I can say very strongly that this need not be true. However, I do feel that girls like Alison need long-term professional therapy, not just drugs and brief hospitalisation, to help them learn to 'feed' themselves – give themselves the things they need, such as food or privacy or rest and relaxation – without feeling guilty, and to recognise what these hungers and desires are.

If reading Alison's story sets off alarm bells in your head about whether you too have an exercise obsession, or perhaps have a friend or sister who does, then turn to 'Obsessions: Where to get help'. Asking yourself the questions Alison suggests can help you to put your own situation into perspective.

How Do I Look?

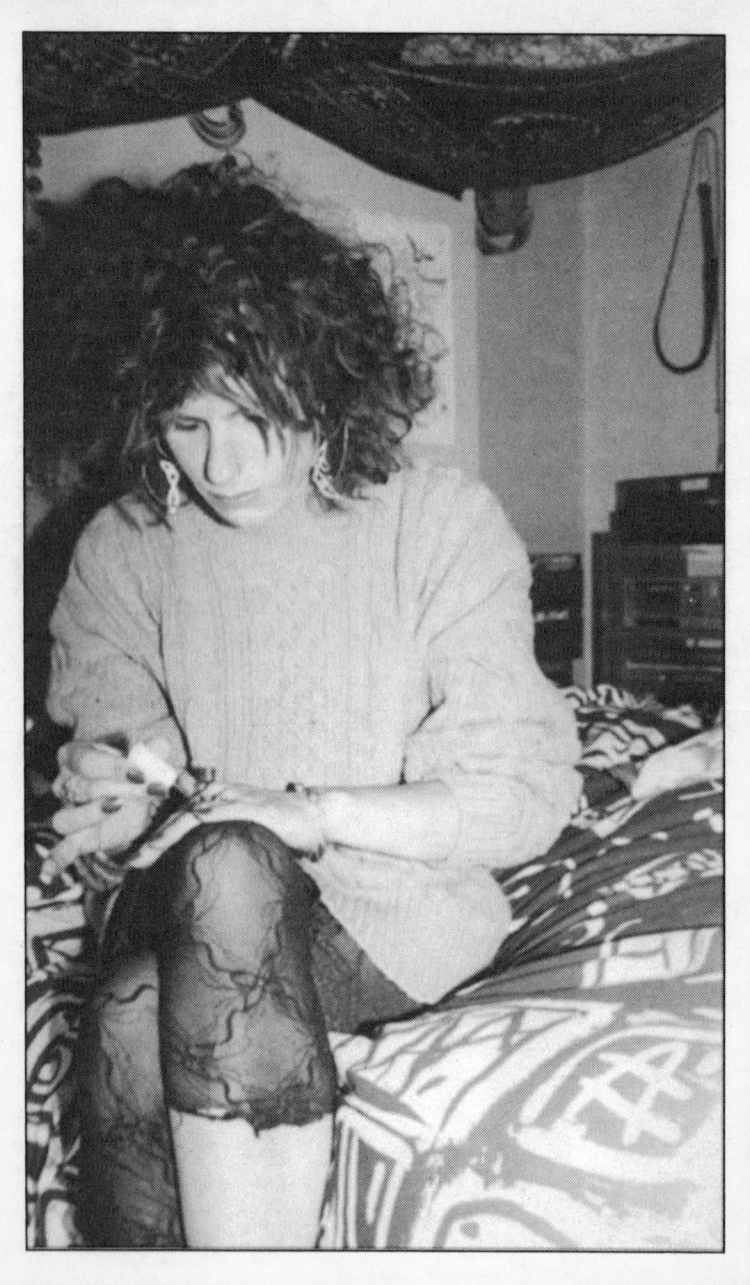

12
Freya

I'M ALWAYS LOOKING AT MYSELF THROUGH OTHER PEOPLE'S EYES

Freya's letter looked as though she had written it in a great hurry: reams and reams of handwritten scrawl, with sentences crawling up the side of the page and ideas jumping all over the place. Mostly she wrote about her feelings about her body and her recent acknowledgement to herself that she was suffering from anorexia. I had the feeling on reading it that a dam had just burst, and that she had a great deal more to say. Freya's confusion and bewilderment are very apparent in this letter, and she gives a sense of having 'fallen into' anorexia, in a strikingly different way to Alison (in the last chapter), who has a much more determined, almost deliberate approach. Since many books that I have read on eating disorders tend to lump all the 'patients' together, ignoring their differences, I thought it might be more useful to let two girls tell their own stories.

Freya thanked me at the end of her letter for 'taking the time to care about a subject so little understood', which was a sentence I heard often from girls in one way or another, in researching this book.

The guilt that girls feel about eating, being fat, or about their bodies in general, and in particular their guilt about what they think of as their 'vanity' if they are obsessed with their bodies, came up over and over again. One girl spent the whole afternoon talking to me about her family's obsession with beauty, how she had always been praised and noticed for being pretty and not much else, and then, just at the end, spoke guiltily of 'wasting my time' with a subject so unimportant. Girls with anorexia or bulimia often feel to blame for their original 'weight problem', then to blame for becoming too obsessed with it, and then further to blame for being unable to 'pull themselves together'. Feelings of guilt are really about a sense of unentitlement; in thinking that your desires and feelings are wrong or 'silly' you are also saying that you feel you are wrong or silly, and not entitled to be taken seriously, or helped.

Freya, like many other girls who wrote to me, mentions her low opinion of herself as leading to, or contributing to, her anorexia. Another girl, Rita, suffering from bulimia, says that 'advertising is not to blame for eating disorders, but can certainly contribute if you have a poor self-image already'. This poor self-image is clearly not just about looks but also about identity and worth – whether you are 'worth anything', whether your problems are serious or important enough to trouble anyone with. This feeling of being worthless is, I think, connected to self-image in the sense that the world tends to measure your worth according to how pretty you are; whether you get a job, a boyfriend, or success in many fields can depend on it. So for girls, worth and beauty are interwoven. Try as we might to tell ourselves that it's 'what's on the inside that counts', we have very little evidence to show that it's true, and inside and outside can become confused, so that we feel bad on the inside but believe that if we altered what's on the outside (our bodies) we could change how we feel.

'The only way I ever look at myself is through other people's eyes. That may sound strange – what I mean is, I'm always trying to imagine what they think of me; I don't seem able to look from inside of myself, outwards. Maybe I don't feel as if I exist in my own right.

I would never, ever have said I was anorexic, until a neighbour and now a close friend, Anita, came out and labelled me one. I was taken aback, but deep down I wasn't totally surprised. I hadn't let myself stop and think about it, but I knew there was something very wrong with me, and although I wasn't depressed exactly, I was going through hell. The reason she said I was anorexic was to do with the proportion of body fat I had lost. Her job is working with girls with eating disorders, so she is very technical about it. I don't think you really need to approach it that way; I think deep down every girl knows herself how serious her own problem is.

About five weeks before that I had come home in my first university term, and got undressed for my bath in front of the bathroom mirror. I looked horrible – this bony, awkward, pitiful image. What really struck me was that I looked like a concentration camp prisoner. I come from a Jewish family which includes victims; that picture of myself was a particularly horrible one. When I saw it, I felt like giving up. I wanted to curl into a tiny ball and be forgotten about by everyone. I would have committed suicide if I could, but I was too scared. What I really would have liked would have been to disappear with as little fuss as possible.

I suppose underneath it was a cry for help. Even now, I'm not sure what it was that I wanted to say, and talking to my new friend is the only way I am learning. She has encouraged me to talk about what happened before I got to that stage, and to think about what might have led up to it.

The whole thing started about a year before, when I was seventeen. I used to be quite big and not exactly overweight, but largeish. I never stopped to think about it, I was used to it. I wished I was prettier in my face sometimes, but nothing much. I had a longstanding boyfriend whom I was happy with. But things started to change when a friend mentioned that since I had lost a little weight whilst being away on a beach holiday with my boyfriend (not deliberately, just through not eating much in the heat of Spain) several people had said how I looked better. For some reason, this really got to me. I felt betrayed; I had never thought of all my friends noticing my weight, and that they had all been thinking of me as a fat person. I was furious, and hurt, but it didn't sink in at first.

What they had said really "took seed" a few months later, when I set off on a world trip for seven months, and during that time the friend I was with, Ella, decided a few times, in different parts of the world, to lose some weight and tone up. I joined her, a bit reluctantly – I would have felt awful not joining in, because I needed it more than she did! She is beautiful and quite sporty. I felt really good a few pounds lighter and with a tan, and I wanted to stay like that and surprise everyone when I got back, especially my boyfriend, who might have been wishing I was thinner. Half of me wanted to "wow" everyone with how good I looked – show them I could do it, be thin if I wanted – but half of me also wanted them not to notice. I wanted it to be that I hadn't really been that big before I left – in other words, prove them wrong.

I still had this idea that my weight was too personal a topic for other people to talk about. People did notice and comment, of course, which embarrassed me. I was in a panic about keeping the weight off, and that's when I think things got serious, particularly when I started my first term at university. I was self-conscious about my body to a painful degree, and terrified lest the weight came back.

My breasts had developed quite early, and although I was proud of them it was also embarrassing, especially at school. My best friends used to twang my bra straps in front of the boys, and although I always laughed, I felt humiliated. The others were pretty and popular, I was trying desperately to fit in with them, but it was dreadful to have something that I was proud of, and happy with – my body – made fun of in that way, by my friends. It really hurt me.

My parents or family had never made a big deal about my body or development. There was no excitement about my first bra – I even had to pay, because my mum claimed I didn't need one! She made me feel happy about having large breasts, because she herself had always wanted them. When I got my period, my family made it a happy, celebratory occasion, in their own way. My dad never talked about appearance much, only to make a clinical/medical-type comment.

My sister always had her own trendy style; ever since we were little I've been aware that she was prettier than me, but she is unassuming and unaware of it. She is a lovely person, it would be hard to feel jealous of her, but I do feel a little envious if I stop to think about it. When we were dressing up as kids, I always tried to look elegant, classy, sexy or feminine, whereas she dressed more how she wanted in weird and wacky costumes, like a cowboy outfit. I half disapproved of these costumes, they made me feel uncomfortable, but at the same time I admired and envied her, she was so original and unconcerned.

Since talking to Anita, my neighbour, about my weight loss and panic about putting it back on, I've discovered what a low opinion I have of myself. A lot of it has been focused on my body – first for being too fat, now for being too thin. I would never try on something revealing like a swimming costume in a communal changing room, because when I was bigger I'd be thinking everyone would be looking at the bulgy bits thinking how fat I was (well, this is what I thought after I found out what my friends had been saying), and now I would feel too self-conscious because other girls would be thinking how skinny I look. The best feeling would be if I could just dismiss everyone else from my mind.

On the other hand, something like walking past a building site in the summer in shorts is *much* easier now that I've lost weight. I feel as if I can slip by, no one will notice me or comment. I was scared of verbal abuse before, when I was bigger; now it's great to feel invisible.

But I am slowly getting better, with Anita's help. This involves putting on weight, but mostly talking. I realise that all this is a jumble, and doesn't explain why my anorexia started, or how it is easing, but this is the stage I'm at right now. Only a few weeks ago I was in such a fog, I wouldn't have been able to write any of this. I haven't had a period for over a year, and although sometimes I think to myself "I'm all right really", then I remember I haven't got my periods back and I realise that it's not as simple as it seems. I think I am just starting out on the steep, rocky – and lots of other corny metaphors – road to recovery.'

Whilst Alison states at the end of Chapter 11 that she would not like to have a period as it would signify that she had 'let up' control over her body, Freya feels quite differently, realising

How Do I Look?

that getting her periods back would be a good sign of recovery. I think that a belief that periods are 'good' and an indicator or product of health and wellbeing is really vital to making a full recovery from any eating disorder which causes your periods to stop, or become irregular. But this, of course, is not simple. How many girls or young women, with or without eating disorders, *do* actually see their periods in this light? Deborah (Chapter 2) mentions how advertising 'pretties up periods', and it is a fact that since putting ads on television for sanitary products, the Independent Broadcasting Authority has had more complaints than for any other product, which says a lot about the public's discomfort and embarrassment where periods are concerned. Despite some changes in our attitudes towards periods they still tend to be seen as at best a nuisance, at worst a painful monthly ordeal.

I remember my own mother saying, when I was undergoing tests to discover why my periods had stopped, that we we needn't worry, they were an expensive nuisance, what did I want periods for anyway? At first glance her remark seems true enough, but my feelings were quite the opposite. Like Freya, I *knew* something was wrong with me precisely because my periods hadn't come back, and weirder still (I thought), I *wanted* them to. Thinking about this now, I know that what I was saying in wanting my periods back was that I wanted to be a woman, that I *wanted* and liked my female body, that my years of confusion and self-dislike were beginning to be over.

It is interesting to me that periods are never seen as *important*. When I tried asking the girls I interviewed about them I was often met with a shrug, or a short 'no problem' reply, as if periods were nothing at all, of no significance, and certainly none to a book on looks, fashion and body-image. But it strikes me that this is really the view of people who don't have them. Without our reproductive system, there would be no life, so they can hardly be unimportant. And something that happens to us at least five days in every month – that affects, amongst other things, our sexual feelings, and our body size and shape – why should that be unimportant?

Deborah, in Chapter 2, talks about the celebration that she

Obsessions

and her family had when she started hers; Deborah has a very good self-image and no particular hang-ups about her body. I think that if periods were seen as something 'natural', 'good' and 'healthy', instead of painful, unclean and embarrassing, then girls and women would feel a lot better about themselves.

Freya's story is unusual in some ways, in that unlike Alison Freya started off, as she says, quite happy with her body; it was the reaction of other people that made her uncertain. I think this is about our physical boundaries again, as it was in Alison's story, showing how fragile the self-image of girls can be, how easily invaded by others – and also, how difficult it is to like your body if it is curvaceous, if you are naturally fleshy, fat, large-breasted or pear-shaped, as many of us are.

Reading Alison and Freya's stories may worry you, puzzle you, or make you wonder whether *your* feelings about your body, or constant dieting or guilt over food, makes *you* obsessive, or verging on an eating disorder. Perhaps you feel that you are not as extreme as either of them, and that may reassure you. But I have deliberately left out in both those chapters the actual details of weight lost or gained, and have done the same in my own story at the beginning of the book. Freya's friend Anita's remark that Freya was anorexic because she had lost a certain amount of body weight is, I feel, misleading, and as Freya rightly points out, she knew herself, deep down, that something was wrong. If you feel constantly anxious and frightened about food, if you cannot take pleasure in eating or in your body, if you know deep down that something is wrong, then it is irrelevant what you weigh or whether your immediate health is at risk; you should take yourself and your feelings seriously, and look for help.

OBSESSIONS: WHERE TO GET HELP; BOOKLIST

Eating Disorders Association: Sackville Place, 44 Magdalen Street, Norwich, Norfolk NR3 1JE (helpline: Mon–Fri 9–4 p.m. 0603 621414) or The Priory Centre, 11 Priory Road, High Wycombe, Bucks HP13 6SL

The Women's Therapy Centre (offers individual or group therapy, unfortunately based only in London and quite expensive, but can put you in touch with a therapist in your area, and offer discounts to unemployed or low-waged): 6 Manor Gardens, London N7 6LA. Telephone: 071 263 6200

Women's Therapy and Counselling Service (drop-in service for girls/women): Oxford Chambers, Oxford Place, Leeds LS1 3AX. Telephone: 0532 455725

Alcohol abuse and eating disorders often go together; they can be symptoms of the same underlying problem. If you feel that your drinking is out of control, you can contact the Women's Alcohol Centre for counselling, support or information: 254 St Paul's Road, London N1 2LJ. Telephone: 071 226 4581

If you think you may be suffering from anorexia, bulimia, compulsive eating or an exercise obsession, you could also try your local doctor, or even a teacher or lecturer at college, and see if s/he could put you in touch with a counsellor or support group in your area.

Booklist

There are many books on the subjects of eating disorders, or body-image and fat hatred. Many, especially those on eating disorders, I have not found particularly helpful, and there are still others that I would positively *not* recommend! In the main I would say these tend to be addressed to parents, doctors or well-meaning teachers, carers, etc., and it is quite difficult to find a book which talks to you, the anorexic/bulimic/compulsive eater. One such is Marilyn Lawrence's *The Anorexic Experience* (The Women's Press, 1984), which I found *did* talk about my experiences without making me feel weirder than ever, or a mere statistic. It may also help if you have an exercise obsession, as Marilyn Lawrence, in my opinion, has the most useful things to say on this subject, too.

It is also extremely difficult to find a book addressed to you if you are one of the younger girls suffering from an eating disorder. There is a section in Sue Sharpe's *Voices from Home* (Virago Upstarts, 1990) that may echo your own feelings, entitled 'Dieting to resist'.

Kim Chernin, in her book *Womansize: The Tyranny of Slenderness* (The Women's Press, 1981) talks about compulsive eating, and the pressure on all of us to be/keep slim. *Fat is a Feminist Issue* by Susie Orbach (Hamlyn, 1978) was revolutionary when it first came out, with its detailed look at what it means to be fat and thin in our society, and to each of us individually. *Fat is a Feminist Issue 2* is a practical handbook and tape for compulsive eaters.

Being Fat is not a Sin, by Shelley Bovey (Pandora 1988) talks about the prejudice and oppression suffered by fat people, particularly women, and about ways to feel good about yourself which don't involve losing weight.

Postscript

In the first draft of this book, I left out any description of the young women speaking, and the introduction to each chapter was only a few lines. But I had the feeling that something was missing. I knew that I was fearful of describing the girls I'd met, because I didn't want to fall into the same traps and judgements we had been talking about; on the other hand, I was not being totally honest in leaving out their descriptions, because in fact how they looked interested me very much.

For each meeting, I dressed up. I told most of the young women on the telephone that I'd be wearing a battered black hat, so that they could find me easily. If asked, I would describe myself as average height, with dyed black hair. On each occasion I took at least half an hour to get ready, chose my clothes carefully, brushed my teeth, put my earrings in, wore bright-red lipstick. And on many of the occasions I had the distinct impression that the girls had dressed up too: one girl wore a big hat, another a beautiful sari in purple and black, another wore DM boots and a big overcoat; many wore make-up, jewellery and perfume.

I rarely made a comment on what someone was wearing; we would sit in a park or café or at home discussing image, beauty, fashion and advertising, and skirt around the more obvious, immediate issues of how we both looked, how we were dressed. I ended up with a lot of material on the pressures, conflicts and obsessions side, and not nearly as much about the pleasures, the fun and creativity of putting looks together, the sensual side to feeling good in what you are wearing, the pleasure of dressing up, or challenging people by dressing down. Yet it was that which struck me more than anything, remaining unspoken (and unwritten) but powerful and obvious: how each young woman chose to express herself and her individuality through how she looked became an essential subtext to the book.

These days the rules are slowly changing. Wearing a miniskirt

Postscript

doesn't mean you're a tart; tracksuits don't necessarily mean you're sporty; dungarees don't make you a feminist; and shaving your legs doesn't mean you're unsussed. A dress can be worn with clumpy men's shoes; tracksuit bottoms and loose tops are comfortable, roomy and worn by either sex; second-hand clothes can be put together with new ones; and very few people believe the laws that fashion writers once laid down, such as "no horizontal stripes or light colours for bigger women". I saw Sybil on "Top of the Pops" the day before I started work on the book and she was wearing a gold bra top, huge fake-gold earrings and black trousers pulled in at the waist. She looked huge, noticeable and fantastic. The following day I asked the young women of an all-girls' school I was visiting if they had seen her, and what they thought. Their reaction was loud and mixed, but they were certainly not uninterested.

So in the final version of this book, I've sketched in how the speaker looks, or else how she describes herself. What each speaker says is half the picture, but now we have the missing part: what she also says through how she chooses to look, to make the picture complete.

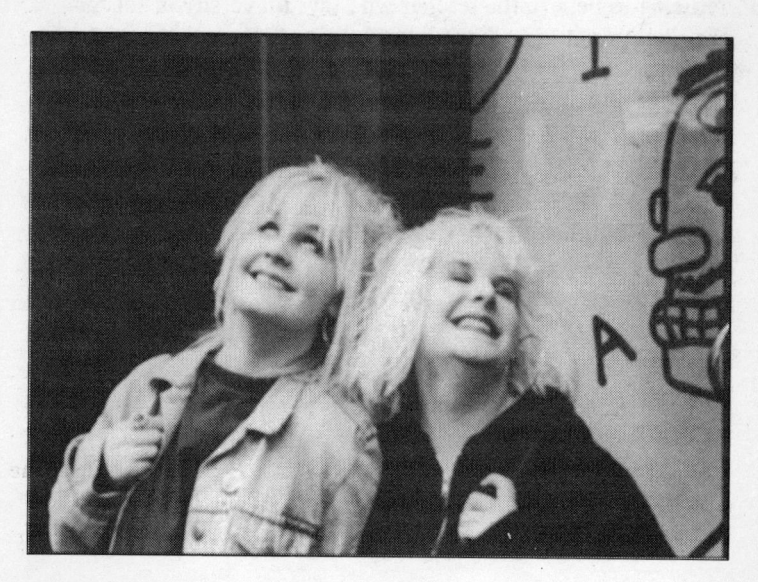

Other Virago Upstarts of interest

TRANSFORMING MOMENTS
Edited by Scarlett MccGwire

'Revelation! It wasn't like a religious experience or anything, significant moments never are. It's that slow dawning of recognition . . .'

Maya Angelou, Melanie McFadyean, Priscilla Presley, Diane Abbott, Eileen Fairweather and Shreela Ghosh, among others, look to their teenage years to find a turning point that altered the course of their lives. What an extraordinary range of stories emerge; first love in a Jewish ghetto; betrayal and expulsion from school; the exhilaration of leaving home; the impact of Jimi Hendrix; teetering on the brink of suicide; refusing to believe the teacher who says university is not for the likes of you. In all our lives are moments or events – dramatic or quiet – that leave us with the certainty that never again will we be quite the same . . .

VOICES FROM HOME
Girls Talk About Their Families

Sue Sharpe

'When I'm older I can be nicer to my parents and do things without having to lie' – Lai

'I remember my dad saying, "Get out of this house, you upset your mum and me so much" ' – Ellie

'I always know they'll stick up for me, whatever. It's something I can't describe, the bond in my family' – Gwyn

Voices From Home explodes the myth of the cosy, happy family into a kaleidoscope of changing patterns. Girls describe their life at home – haven or hell, or both. Here closeness and security jostle with violence and abuse. These are real families – some together, some apart – and no matter what shape it takes, for most girls, family life still pivots around a powerful sense of love and loyalty.

MISFITS AND REBELS
Jenny Oldfield

'I know I should've moved on. It's no good getting to like people. But this time I wasn't looking. She seeped in like those oil stains in the garage'

Life on the edge, where dangerous emotions – anger, fear and longing – lurk just beneath the surface. There's Stuart, on the run; Maddie, mad by name and mad by nature; Sam, brown and fast as the wind; Siobhan, fiercely guarding her love for her mother. Do you take a risk and try to find something roughly called happiness, or do you take lonely refuge in being on the outside? Bold and urgent, this string of stories is about kids who find their own view of the world and their own place in it.

UP THE ATTIC STAIRS
Angela Bull

'I've been visiting Springfield to look at the clothes . . . I was finding out about our family – it's fascinating. Except we're all doomed'

Curiosity and troubles draw fashion student Gabriel back home to Springfield and up the attic stairs. There she rediscovers Victorian dresses, Edwardian hats crowned with crimson roses, 1920s cocktail frocks – and a journal about her family. She begins to unravel a past filled with suffragettes and spinsters; balls and dress shops; a house of women who harbour an illegitimate baby girl during the Second World War; and much disappointed love . . . I, too, am ill-fated in love and life, despairs Gabriel. But has she really understood her ancestors' lives?

NELL'S QUILT
Susan Terris

' "I will marry Anson Tanner!" Even as the delaration escaped from my mouth, I knew I wished to suck it back in and chew it to shreds. But I couldn't. Once I gave my word about something, I kept it'

When eighteen-year-old Nell finally agrees to marry the widower her parents have chosen for her, it means she must give up her dreams of going to college and following in her suffragist grandmother's footsteps. That spring day, in 1899, she virtually stops eating and begins to piece and embroider a quilt. As it grows ever larger and more magnificent, Nell, almost imperceptibly, grows frailer and weaker and not very interested in the real world anymore . . .